Inpatient Psychiatric Nursing

Linda Damon, MSN, MHA, RN, is the vice president of patient care services, Butler Hospital, Providence, RI, where she is responsible for the quality of nursing care and operations of inpatient, partial hospital services, and admission services in a 147-bed hospital. She has held senior management positions at Cambridge Health Alliance Department of Psychiatry (Cambridge, MA); Horizon Health Corporation, provider of psychiatric management services (Lewisville, TX); and McLean Hospital, a private Harvard-affiliated psychiatric hospital (Belmont, MA). In addition, she has served as adjunct faculty at the Community College of RI (Providence, RI), MGH Institute for Health Professionals, Boston College (Boston, MA), and the University of Massachusetts Lowell (Lowell, MA). Her professional affiliations include membership in the American Nurses Association (member delegate from RI '08 and '10), Rhode Island State Nurses Association (RISNA) American Psychiatric Nurses Association (APNA) Massachusetts Organization of Nurse Executives (MONE), American Organization of Nurse Executives (AONE), and the RI Board of Registration in Nursing.

Joanne M. Matthew, MSN, PMHCNS-BC, RN, is a nurse manager in adult intensive treatment unit at Butler Hospital, Providence, RI. She also serves as clinical instructor in psychiatric mental health nursing at the University of Rhode Island, School of Nursing. She is a member of the APNA Administrative Steering Council and a task force member of the APNA Institute for Safe Environments: Physiological Risks of Restraint and Seclusion (2009).

Judy L. Sheehan, MSN, RN, is the director of nursing education at Butler Hospital, Providence, RI. She also serves as the nurse peer review leader for the Massachusetts Association of Registered Nurses, Committee of Continuing Education and is a clinical instructor in psychiatric nursing at the University of Rhode Island College of Nursing. In addition, she has served as adjunct faculty for Salve Regina University and the Massachusetts School of Pharmacy and Allied Health. Her professional affiliations include membership in the American Psychiatric Nurses Association, The National Nurses in Staff Development Organization and the American Nurses Association. Ms. Sheehan has contributed to two books and published the CD-ROM *De-Stress: Coping and Managing Computer Generated Stress.*

Lisa A. Uebelacker, PhD, holds multiple appointments including staff psychologist at Butler Hospital, Providence, RI; affiliate staff, Department of Family Medicine at Memorial hospital, Pawtucket, RI; and assistant professor, Department of Psychology and Human Behavior at Brown University, Providence, RI. She serves as an ad hoc reviewer for many psychology journals and is on the editorial board of the *Journal of Family Psychology.* Dr. Uebelacker has published more than 45 peer-reviewed articles. She has also been the principal investigator or co-principal investigator on 10 funded research grants.

Inpatient Psychiatric Nursing

Clinical Strategies & Practical Interventions

Linda Damon, MSN, MHA, RN

Joanne M. Matthew, MSN, PMHCNS-BC, RN

Judy L. Sheehan, MSN, RN

Lisa A. Uebelacker, PhD

Published in cooperation with
Butler Hospital
Providence, Rhode Island
www.butler.org

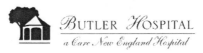

BUTLER HOSPITAL
a Care New England Hospital

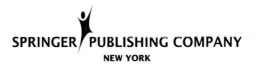

SPRINGER PUBLISHING COMPANY
NEW YORK

Springer Publishing Company, LLC
11 West 42nd Street
New York, NY 10036
www.springerpub.com

Acquisitions Editor: Margaret Zuccarini
Production Editor: Michael O'Connor
Composition: Newgen Imaging

ISBN: 978-0-8261-0971-2
E-book ISBN: 978-0-8261-0972-9

12 13 14 15 / 5 4 3 2

The author and the publisher of this Work have made every effort to use sources believed to be reliable to provide information that is accurate and compatible with the standards generally accepted at the time of publication. Because medical science is continually advancing, our knowledge base continues to expand. Therefore, as new information becomes available, changes in procedures become necessary. We recommend that the reader always consult current research, specific institutional policies, and current drug references before performing any clinical procedure or administering any drug. The author and publisher shall not be liable for any special, consequential, or exemplary damages resulting, in whole or in part, from the readers' use of, or reliance on, the information contained in this book. The publisher has no responsibility for the persistence or accuracy of URLs for external or third-party Internet Web sites referred to in this publication and does not guarantee that any content on such Web sites is, or will remain, accurate or appropriate.

Library of Congress Cataloging-in-Publication Data
Inpatient psychiatric nursing : clinical strategies & practical interventions / [edited by] Linda Damon ... [et al.].
  p. ; cm.
Includes bibliographical references and index.
ISBN 978-0-8261-0971-2—ISBN 978-0-8261-0972-9 (e-book)
I. Damon, Linda, RN.
  [DNLM: 1. Mental Disorders—nursing. 2. Mental Disorders—therapy. 3. Psychiatric Nursing—methods. WY 160]
LC classification not assigned
616.89'0231—dc23   2012006971

Printed in the United States of America by Gasch Printing

This book is dedicated to psychiatric nurses, past, present and future and the patients they serve.

Contents

Contributors

Cynthia Belonick, APRN-BC
Nurse Educator
The Institute of Living,
   Hartford, Connecticut

Ellen Blair, APRN-BC
Director of Nursing
The Institute of Living,
   Hartford, Connecticut

**Barbara-Ann Bybel,
   DHA, MSN, NEA-BC,
   PMHNP-BC**
Patient Care Director
New York Presbyterian
   Hospital, New York

**Linda Damon, MSN,
   MHA, RN**
Vice President of Patient Care
   Services, Chief Nursing
   Officer
Butler Hospital, Providence,
   Rhode Island

Maryann DaSilva, BSN, RN
Nurse Manager of Adult
   Services, D3
Butler Hospital, Providence,
   Rhode Island

Laura Drury, MSW, LICSW
Clinical Director of Social Work
Butler Hospital, Providence,
   Rhode Island

**Mary E. Dubreuil, RN, MA
(2012) LCDP**
Director of Alcohol and Drug
   Treatment Services
Butler Hospital, Providence,
   Rhode Island

Nancy Egan, RN, MEd
Nurse Manger, Child and
   Adolescent Treatment
   Services
Butler Hospital, Providence,
   Rhode Island

Linda Espinosa, MS, RN
Vice President of Patient
   Care Services
New York Presbyterian
   Hospital, New York

Diane Ferreira, RN, MHA
Director of Social Services
Butler Hospital, Providence,
   Rhode Island

Nicole Flanagan, BA, BSN, RN
Nurse Manager of Adult
    Services, D4
Butler Hospital, Providence,
    Rhode Island

**Judith L. Giorgi-Cipriano,
    MS, RN**
Director of Quality and
    Patient Services
New York Presbyterian
    Hospital, New York

**Elizabeth Harris, RN, MA,
    PMHCNS-BC**
Health Education Coordinator
New York Presbyterian
    Hospital, New York

**Debora Heidtman,
    RN, MHA**
Director of Adult Services and
    Kent Unit
Butler Hospital, Providence,
    Rhode Island

Susan Higgins, MA, OTR/L
Occupational Therapist
Butler Hospital, Providence,
    Rhode Island

Joan S. Kovach, RN, MS, PC
Nurse Director
McLean Hospital, South East
    Unit
McLean Hospital, Belmont
Massachusetts

Karen Larsen, RN-BC
RN Clinical Coordinator
The Institute of Living,
    Hartford, Connecticut

**Mary Leveillee, PhD(c), RN
    PCNS, MS**
Director, Undergraduate
    Program
College of Nursing
University of Rhode Island
Rhode Island

Angela Macera, RN, MBA, BS
Patient Care Director
New York Presbyterian
    Hospital, New York

**Joanne M. Matthew, MSN,
    PMHCNS-BC, RN**
Director of Nursing Quality
    and Intensive Treatment
    Unit
Butler Hospital, Providence,
    Rhode Island

Emily McCue, BSN RN
Staff Nurse, Kent Unit
Butler Hospital, Providence,
    Rhode Island

**Julie Armstrong Muth, MS,
    RN, NE, BC**
Director of Nursing and
    Quality
New York Presbyterian
    Hospital, New York

Barbara Ostrove, MA, OTR/L
Director of Occupational
    Therapy
Butler Hospital, Providence,
    Rhode Island

Christopher Paiva, RN-BC, BSN
Nursing Director of the Behavioral Health Unit
Newport Hospital, Newport, Rhode Island

Michelle Pereira, RN, MHA
Director of Risk management and Business Development
Butler Hospital, Providence, Rhode Island

Idrialis Perez, RN, BSN
Clinical Assistant Nurse Manager, Senior Specialty Unit
Butler Hospital, Providence, Rhode Island

Patricia R. Recupero, JD, MD
Board Certified in Addictions and Forensic Psychiatry
President/CEO, Butler Hospital, Providence, Rhode Island

Kevin Ritchie, RN, BSN
Staff Nurse, Kent Unit
Butler Hospital, Providence, Rhode Island

Kristen Sayles, BA, BS, RN
Clinical Assistant Nurse Manager, Kent Unit
Butler Hospital, Providence, Rhode Island

Judy L. Sheehan, MSN, RN
Director of Nursing Education
Butler Hospital, Providence, Rhode Island

Debra Spellman, BSN, RN
Staff Nurse, Kent Unit
Butler Hospital, Providence, Rhode Island

Kristi Svendsen, RN, MA, CAGS, LCDP
Clinical Assistant Nurse Manager, Alcohol and Drug Treatment Unit
Butler Hospital, Providence, Rhode Island

Mary Trainor, RN, BSN
Staff Nurse, Senior Specialty Unit
Butler Hospital, Providence, Rhode Island

Christopher Towey, RN, BA
Clinical Assistant Nurse Manager, Intensive Treatment Unit
Butler Hospital, Providence, Rhode Island

Lisa A. Uebelacker, PhD
Research Psychologist
Butler Hospital, Providence, Rhode Island, Alpert Medical School of Brown University

Preface

Due to a changing health care landscape, inpatient psychiatric nursing practice has changed dramatically over the past decades. The patients who now receive care in an acute care setting have to be very ill and typically exhibit considerable behavioral impairments and multiple safety concerns. The average length of stay is often between 5 and 10 days, and the resources available to these patients after discharge vary considerably depending upon their own health insurance and the community from which they come. Psychiatric nurses who practice in the inpatient acute care setting find themselves challenged by a wide range of patient symptoms and behaviors that occur in the context of the complex and ever-changing treatment environment on the psychiatric unit. As we read the psychiatric nursing literature, we found that many authors focused extensively on treatment of specific diagnoses. Yet, a group of individuals with a given diagnosis are often very heterogeneous and exhibit many different types of behaviors. In the psychiatric nursing literature, there was much less information on managing specific *behaviors* (which may be transdiagnostic) on an acute inpatient unit. Therefore, we wanted to share our insights on the many approaches to managing the specific behaviors that psychiatric nurses see on an inpatient unit every day. This book primarily includes *practice-based evidence*. Wherever possible, we also tried to place our own practical experiences in the context of current literature and research.

Inpatient Psychiatric Nursing: Clinical Strategies and Practical Interventions is a handbook for psychiatric nurses, nursing students, new nurses, or other nurses who are new to working with patients having psychiatric conditions. In this handbook, we describe specific aspects of inpatient psychiatric nursing practice, with a focus on three types of inpatient treatment goals: keeping the patient safe, stabilizing symptoms, and promoting engagement in treatment. A fourth goal is discharge planning. This book is organized according to patient behaviors (Part I) and interventions that nurses can employ to manage behaviors (Part II). In Part I, there is a consistent chapter format so that specific content is easy to access, and each chapter concludes with a comprehensive table covering goals, areas of assessment, and interventions of the chapter's covered behavior. (A PDF combining all ten of these tables is available for free download and convenient printing at springerpub.com/ Damon.)

This book grew from a forum of Butler Hospital nurses who came together over a 2-year period to identify and describe successful interventions used in the inpatient psychiatric setting. Feedback from nursing students, new graduate nurses, and newly employed nurses on the inpatient units underscored the need for such a resource. *Clinical Strategies and Practical Interventions* represents a collaboration of the original nurses from Butler Hospital with colleagues from University of Rhode Island, McLean Hospital, New York Presbyterian, and Institute of Living.

Acknowledgments

This book is the result of extensive contributions by the many nurse authors listed on the chapters. Without all their hard work, this would not have been possible. The idea for this book originated with a group of nurses at Butler Hospital who formed a task force that documented the many nursing interventions used with our psychiatrically complex patients. These nurses built the foundation from which we all worked. I am very grateful to this team: Joanne Matthew, Maryann DaSilva, Christopher Paiva, Kristen Sayles, Janet Gould, Sherrill Magnan, Idrialis Perez, Ruth Reavey, Debra Spellman, Karen Tamburro, and Mary Trainor.

I have been blessed to work on this endeavor with such an extraordinary team both at Butler Hospital and at other Ivy League Hospitals, including the Institute of Living, New York Presbyterian, McLean Hospital, and the University of Rhode Island. Without their labor of love, this would not have been accomplished.

I give special thanks to Patricia R. Recupero, MD, JD, President and CEO of Butler Hospital. She encouraged and supported our work. She knew the importance of writing down our successful interventions so that others could learn from them. I also thank Dr. Steve Rasmussen, Medical Director at Butler Hospital, for facilitating my introduction to Lisa A. Uebelacker, PhD, researcher. We, as nurse authors, are forever indebted to Dr. Uebelacker for her collaboration with us. She has been a mentor, teacher, and friend. In addition, I thank my coeditors,

Judy L. Sheehan and Joanne M. Matthew, for their devotion, dedication, and determination in ensuring the work gets done. I also thank my assistant, Geralyn Gabriel, whose attention to detail and organization allow us all to succeed.

Lastly, I thank each and every nurse who cares for patients with psychiatric illness. Your work is challenging, your commitment inspiring!

Linda Damon, MSN, MHA, RN

The Patient With Anger

1

*Joanne M. Matthew, Kristen Sayles,
and Maryann DaSilva*

BACKGROUND AND DESCRIPTION

Anger is a basic human emotion that is normal and expected under certain situations. Anger serves as an energizing function that enables an individual to act on perceived threats (Novaco, 1976). However, the individual's expression of anger or behavior when angry can become a problem for the individual and others. Some individuals escalate quickly from annoyance or frustration to rage and may have a reduced ability to exercise control over their angry responses (Murphy & Carsen, 2010). In fact, individuals who are quick to anger may have more sensitive or dysfunctional central nervous system, which governs wakefulness and vigilance; these individuals are highly alert to potential threats and consequently respond rapidly to perceived threats (Murphy & Carsen, 2010; Perry & Szalavitz, 2006). Research demonstrates that individuals with high levels of anger arousal are at risk for violent behaviors and cardiovascular diseases (Murphy & Carsen, 2010; Novaco, 2007.)

Anger can be distinguished from aggression, which is a physical or verbal action of directed harm to objects or others (Hollinworth, Clark, Harland, Johnson, & Partington, 2005; Murphy & Carsen, 2010; Thomas, 2001). In this chapter, we focus on early identification of anger and preventative interventions to interrupt the escalation of anger to aggressive or violent behaviors.

Behavior

Some of the behaviors associated with anger are a reflection of a patient's state of physical arousal. During the early phase of anger, the patient may be quieter but will still demonstrate identifiable body language and behaviors, such as turning away from a group, muttering, or beginning to make hostile comments to staff and peers. Her face may redden, and her fists or jaw may clench. Sometimes, the individuals' actions may not be notable, but the way that they change positions more abruptly, move quickly, or act more forcefully will provide some indication of a changing emotional state from mild annoyance or irritation to anger.

In contrast, sometimes the angry patient is easy to identify, as he will be very active, may pace back and forth, and have trouble sitting still. This individual may speak loudly, often in clipped tones or in a rapid manner, while making wild gestures, poking a finger at others, or shaking his fists. The angry patient may begin to stomp his feet, slam doors, or put down a magazine or other object with more force than is required.

The emotion of anger is thought to be experienced similarly across gender although the expression of anger is modified by social roles (Fischer, Mosquera, Van Vianen, & Manstead, 2004). Beliefs about proper expression of anger can be different for cultures considered to be more individualistic (e.g., the United States) compared with more collectivistic cultures (e.g., Japan). In a collectivistic culture, the expression of anger may be seen as a threat to the important value of harmony in relationships and therefore individuals may try to suppress overt signs of anger. In contrast, an individualistic culture will value socially appropriate expressions of anger as being needed to protect individual rights and freedom (Hollinworth, et al., 2005). However, because there can be a wide range of behaviors and attitudes within any given cultural group, it is important to consider each patient individually when assessing ability to manage angry feelings.

With regard to gender differences, there are inconsistencies in the body of literature that examines gender differences in emotions and the expression of emotion (Cheung & Park, 2010; Fischer, et al., 2004). Some studies have found that anger is more often outwardly expressed by men than women; however, these differences may be less distinct in some cultural groups (Safdar et al., 2009). Further, across genders, the trait of expressing anger outwardly is associated with increased cardiovascular risk factors.

Cognition

An individual's appraisal of a situation, as well as her expectations for what should occur, can lead to anger. Anger is often a response to a perceived injustice, a perceived disrespect, a personal insult, or a physical threat to personal safety (Hollinworth et al. 2005; Murphy & Carsen, 2010). A patient who is angry may believe she has been mistreated or treated unfairly. Another individual may feel trapped, that she has no choices, or that she must defend herself. Sometimes the trigger to the angry response is not clear to the staff or the individual.

Angry behavior can be fueled by certain beliefs about anger. For example, an individual may be thinking, "No one listens to me unless I yell," or "no one respects me" (Murphy & Carsen, 2010). Another person who is distressed by his anger may believe "I shouldn't feel like this about someone," or "I am not a good person if I feel this way."

When a person is extremely angry, cognitive processes may be impaired. The individual may act before evaluating the consequences of his actions. In addition, the individual may have difficulty reflecting on his behavior or processing multiple or complex instructions or requests (Murphy & Carsen, 2010; Novaco, 1976).

Affect

Anger is a natural human emotion and can serve as an adaptive function, such as a signal that there is a problem in the individual's environment. The expression of anger occurs on a spectrum of emotion from mild annoyance or irritation to frustration or anger and to rage and possibly aggression (Murphy & Carsen, 2010). For some individuals, feelings of vulnerability, sadness, shame, or fear can lead to anger (Davila, 1999; Tangney, Wagner, Fletcher, & Gramzow, 1992). The individual's experience of anger can be extreme and personally distressing. For some, anxiety and guilt may occur in response to feeling angry (Thomas, 2001).

Context

Difficulty coping with anger and rapid escalation to rage or aggression sometimes occurs in individuals with psychiatric diagnoses such as bipolar disorder, posttraumatic stress disorder (PTSD), substance abuse or dependence, major depression, and personality disorders, especially Cluster B (Murphy & Carsen, 2010; Novaco, 2007). An acute exacerbation of these conditions can make angry feelings and behaviors even more difficult to manage. Individuals who have a medical condition that decreases their ability to regulate their emotions or increases their impulsivity, such as stroke or traumatic brain injury (TBI), could also have problems coping with anger (Murphy & Carsen, 2010; Quanbeck & McDermott, 2008).

There are other contexts for anger as a problem as well. Individuals who have few positive coping skills or who have experienced childhood neglect or trauma may have problems managing their emotions, including anger (Murphy & Carsen, 2010). Anger can be a stage in the grief process, and patients who have experienced multiple losses or one significant loss may experience anger. Some individuals may have frequent angry responses on the inpatient unit, in part, because it is a restrictive, highly regimented, and controlled setting (Murphy & Carsen, 2010).

Finally, there is a Korean anger disorder called "hwa-byung." The development of this disorder is ascribed to long-term suppression of anger that accumulates and results in symptoms of feeling angry, expressing anger, feeling physical sensations of heat, and feelings of hate. It is found in 4.1% of the Korean population, most often in middle-age or older women (Min & Suh, 2010).

POTENTIAL BARRIERS TO BEING THERAPEUTIC

Witnessing angry acts or being subjected to the angry venting of a patient can bring up feelings of fear, anger, helplessness, or anxiety in a nurse. Depending on the nurse's own experiences and way of handling anger, he may feel angry toward the patient. This may cause the nurse to respond punitively to this patient. The nurse who feels fearful may avoid the patient, thus hesitating to intervene early or effectively. Finally, when angry patients make threats against the nurse and challenge her competence and livelihood, the nurse may respond defensively or hesitantly as she may begin to doubt herself. As is often the challenge with patients, the nurse must understand her own responses to anger and aggression and use that understanding to be able to respond in a therapeutic way (Murphy & Carsen, 2010).

OVERVIEW OF NURSING CARE GOALS

1. **Safety**
   - Prevent or reduce the risk for harm to others
2. **Stabilization**
   - Increase anger management skills
3. **Engagement**
   - Increase engagement in treatment

SAFETY

● **Subgoal: Prevent or Reduce Risk for Harm to Others**

Assessment of Risk for Harm to Others

Angry patients who are in a rage present a risk for violence to others. Sometimes, this risk is the result of a direct assault. Other times, it will be inadvertent due to the patient throwing objects during an angry outburst. In this chapter, we focus on assessment and interventions that can prevent the patient progressing to this stage.

In report. The nurse will listen for specific indications that the patient has a problem with anger and/or has been violent in the past. Consequently, the circumstances of the admission, history of violence, and diagnosis are all important. Is the patient here involuntarily? Has he assaulted anyone recently or in the past? Is there any history of domestic violence, childhood abuse, or neglect? (Murphy & Carsen, 2010). The nurse will also listen for any assessment ratings that indicate anger escalation or aggression risk (see *"On the unit"* below). The nurse will consider whether the angry aggression is related to an acute stressor or a more permanent change in behavior. For example, is the anger or irritability related to a bipolar episode, and might the anger resolve as the episode resolves? Is the patient chronically and emotionally dysregulated, such as someone with

PTSD or a personality disorder? Is the patient intoxicated or does she have a history of a TBI? The nurse's knowledge and understanding of the nature and chronicity of anger problems will serve to guide intervention. In some cases, treatment or resolution of the underlying problem (e.g., intoxication) will be sufficient to manage anger and prevent aggression. In other cases, when the underlying problem is more chronic, as in TBI, anger may be a problem throughout the entire hospital stay and require active management.

One-to-one contact. During the initial nursing assessment, the nurse will want to ascertain the patient's perception of why she is in the hospital. The nurse may ask, "Can you tell me why you are here?" "What are your goals for hospitalization?" or perhaps, "How can we help you?" If the patient can answer these questions, this is an indication that the patient is able to engage with the nurse further to develop de-escalation preferences or an initial crisis plan for coping with anger and preventing aggression. A wellness assessment or sensory assessment can also provide information about any antecedents to anger, the patient's preferences regarding how to approach him when he is getting angry, and things that may help him calm down, such as talking to staff or being alone. Alternatively, the nurse can ask the patient, "What helps you when you feel angry?" "What should we know about you to help you if you feel angry?" "How do you relax or calm down when you get upset?" The patient may be able to give the nurse important information about how to help her avoid aggressive behavior.

If the patient responds to initial questions with a comment such as "Nothing. I do not belong here," it could indicate an increased risk for aggression because the patient has limited insight or is angry about being hospitalized. Difficulty participating in this initial one-to-one assessment, a hostile attitude, or an irritable mood increases the risk for aggression (Quanbeck & McDermott, 2008).

On the unit. The nurse will want to watch for any physiological signs of arousal in the patient, such as increased muscle tension, increased activity, or increased volume or tone during interactions. In addition, there are particular time periods that involve environmental risk factors that may increase stress and the risk of escalating anger for patients. These periods include shift changes, meals, medication administration times, visiting times, or times when the unit schedule is disrupted (Quanbeck & McDermott, 2008). The nurse will want to monitor patients who have difficulty during these times.

The Broset Violence Checklist (BVC) is a recommended assessment tool that was empirically developed using inpatient chart reviews (Almvik & Woods, 1999). In this scale, a staff is asked to rate whether a patient has been confused, irritable, boisterous, physically threatening, verbally threatening, or attacking objects. The staff rates at a specified time during the working shift. Patients receive one point for each behavior. A total score of 0 represents low risk for violent behavior; a score of 1 or 2 represents a moderate risk; and a score greater than 2 represents a high risk (Almvik & Woods, 1999). Rating the BVC allows the nurse to determine quickly who may be at high risk for violence on the next shift (Abderhalden, Needham, Miserez, Almvik, Dassen, Haug & Fisher, 2004; Almvik & Woods, 1999; Almvik, Woods, & Rasmussen, 2000; Woods, Ashley, Kayto, & Heusdens, 2008).

● Key Nursing Interventions to Reduce Risk of Aggression Toward Others

Three essential nursing interventions for reducing the risk of angry patients acting aggressively are having a plan, managing environmental triggers, and de-escalating the patients (Murphy & Carsen, 2010). The specificity of the plan and the degree to which environmental triggers must be managed will depend upon the likelihood that a patient will become aggressive and the likelihood that the patient will be able to de-escalate. If the nurse believes it will be difficult for the patient to de-escalate, the first two interventions (having a plan and managing environmental triggers) increase in importance.

Have a plan for preventing aggression. The nurse's assessment of the patient's current condition and history, his ability to engage in problem solving, and the assessment of his triggers to anger and skills for coping with anger provides the information that is used to develop a plan for the patient. The purpose of the plan is to prevent aggression. When a patient has been learning about coping skills, he may be able to develop a plan easily with support from the nurse. The nurse and the patient will want to discuss what "the plan" may be around an identified trigger or a difficult time. For example, if the patient has identified that raising his voice is an early sign of escalation, and that this typically happens during group, then the plan may be to have the patient and the group leader decide upon a signal for the patient to leave the group. The patient agrees to leave the group when given this signal. Alternatively, the nurse and the patient may agree that when he shows signs of becoming angry, the nurse or group leader will remind him to come out of group and choose something to help him calm down and refocus.

On some occasions, staff may anticipate the patient responding with anger and possibly aggression to a visitor, the physician, or an outside agency coming to give the patient difficult news. Even if the patient may not be aware of the fact that difficult news is forthcoming, the nurse may make a plan to have extra support for the patient, offer prn medications, and/or have the meeting in a designated safer place on the unit. The nurse's choice of plan will depend on what has worked for this individual in the past. In addition, staff and the patient may anticipate a trigger for aggression during a routine family visit, family meeting, or physician meeting. Together, the nurse and patient can discuss coping alternatives ahead of time and role-play any anticipated difficult moments. In addition, there may be a plan to provide the patient with support after the meeting.

Manage environmental triggers. For the patient who has a brain injury or is intoxicated or manic, the nurse will largely make the plan and manage environmental triggers as well as possible, potentially with minimal input from the patient. Based on her observations and the patient's history, the nurse will attempt to minimize unnecessary exposure to triggers for anger or aggression. The nurse must consider the level of noise and activity on the unit at various times. Increased activity such as multiple new admissions or discharges, visiting times, or large group activities may be triggers for certain patients. Consequently, the nurse will want to consider the room assignment, location, and choice of roommate for this patient. The nurse will also want to guide the patient toward appropriate group or independent activities and potentially remove him from areas of the unit that the nurse expects to get noisy or active in the near future.

Help the patient to de-escalate when needed. De-escalation is needed as early as possible whenever there is indication that a patient is becoming more anxious, angry, or agitated. Early identification of an individual who is becoming angry is important so that the patient and nurse are able to communicate effectively. When the patient is in acute crisis, it is important to remember that she may have a decreased ability to think and communicate clearly.

De-escalation is the process of helping the patient to a "calmer space." It involves respecting the patient, expressing concern for him, validating his feelings, and giving him a choice (Johnson & Hauser, 2001). The majority of patients will respond to de-escalation as long as it is individualized for their needs and preferences. This is the intervention that is useful in all situations regardless of the patient's diagnosis. We describe each of these steps in more detail next.

First, regardless of the whether the patient is in an acute crisis, patients often say that the best nurses treat them like "human beings," or with respect and dignity. Nurses who are successful in de-escalation first ask if they can approach or talk to the patient (Johnson & Hauser, 2001). Second, the nurse validates the patient's feelings of anger, unfairness, or frustration and acknowledges the patient's right to be angry (Hollinworth et al., 2005; Murphy & Carsen, 2010). For example, the nurse may say, "It makes sense that you feel this way." The nurse should also apologize if the situation calls for that. The nurse should not become defensive or make statements about "being too busy." At this point, it will also be helpful for the nurse to assess what may be causing the patient's anger, and whether there is also sadness, fear, or shame. For example, consider the patient who is stating that he is going to "get out of here no matter what." He is demanding to be discharged. Instead of immediately stating what cannot be done, the nurse should genuinely respond to the patient's distress. Is he fearful? Has he given any sign that he is feeling trapped or his anger has been triggered by something? Sometimes, the patient can verbalize these thoughts or feelings. The nurse should look beyond the patient's angry words and try to express to the patient that she can see that he is feeling upset or feeling bad. This can be followed with an expression of wanting to help and an offer of what *can* be done. This is the time to offer a chance to talk, medications, or a call to the patient's physician to address some aspects of what the patient is experiencing.

Third, depending on the situation, the nurse tries to help the patient regain control of his feelings so that he does not escalate into rage or aggression. This is the time to offer the patient choices regarding what to do next, to avoid power struggles with him over inconsequential things, and to allow the patient to exit the situation with his dignity intact and to "save face." This may involve bargaining and compromise (Hollinworth et al., 2005; Lowe, 1992; Murphy & Carsen, 2010). Sometimes, the nurse cannot meet the patient's demand (e.g., to leave the unit immediately) but can offer another solution (e.g., "I will be sure to let the doctor know how you feel"). Sometimes, the patient may identify something that the nurse *can* change. For example, perhaps the patient wants a different roommate or wants to make a phone call. If there is a request that the nurse can accommodate, it may help the patient tolerate denial of other requests.

This is a good time for the nurse to remember that frustration with the rules, restrictions of the setting, or some disappointing news or situation may have triggered anger for this individual. This may help increase the nurse's empathy and enable the nurse to behave flexibly. The nurse will want to take care not to say things that come across as shaming or blaming as this may intensify the patient's anger. This is not a good time to remind the patient of "the rules." For example, many units have a rule that swearing or cursing is not allowed. Instead of saying "watch your language" or "we do not allow swearing here," the nurse might say, "I know that you are upset (or really angry), but I am having trouble hearing you when you swear at me (or yell at me). What you have to say is important." Sometimes, it is effective for the nurse to say that she does not want to fight with the patient; she just wants to help.

STABILIZATION

● Subgoal: Increase Anger Management Skills

Assessment of Readiness for Anger Management Skills and Triggers for Anger
In report. The patient who has reported poor insight and judgment, is hospitalized against her will, or is actively

intoxicated or manic may not have any insight regarding her problems with anger and may not be ready to participate in a discussion of anger management skills (Murphy & Carsen, 2010; Thomas, 2001). This may change over the course of her time on the unit.

The observations heard in report will indicate areas the nurse needs to assess further during one-to-one contact. For example, if the patient has reported homicidal ideation that is not related to a delusional or psychotic process, the nurse will ask the patient more specific questions during their one-to-one contact and assess the patient's willingness to learn new skills to cope with it.

In report, the nurse will want to listen for specific times or situations that may have triggered a reported angry outburst. Does the patient tend to become angry during medication administration times, visiting time, or meal times? The context of the angry outburst may be a clue to a potential trigger such as the denial of a request or the wait time after a request. The nurse can then ask the patient about the trigger and about the patient's interest in learning new coping skills to manage that trigger.

One-to-one contact. The nurse will want to assess the patient's understanding about anger, his perceptions of his angry behavior, and his readiness to learn new skills. Does the patient make statements regarding his angry behavior that place all the blame on others? Is he rationalizing or justifying his behavior? If the patient blames others for "making me angry" or insists that he would not get angry if people did not do certain things, then he may not be ready to participate in a discussion regarding his part in the escalation of anger and how he might better manage angry feelings. For example, consider the patient who is admitted after destroying property in reaction to a spouse's infidelity. She may see her behavior as justified and not problematic.

In addition, patients who demonstrate no distress over their "angry" behavior may not be ready to try to change it or manage it. Finally, the patient who is demonstrating overt signs of angry behavior, such as yelling or slamming doors, but when asked, states that she is not angry at all is likely not ready to consider other ways of responding to angry feelings.

Alternatively, some patients will express regret and say that they wish that they could cope better. They may want to learn new coping skills. Patients who are able to discuss their feelings, their thoughts, and possible triggers to anger will be more likely to be able to learn and practice anger management techniques.

On the unit. The nurses will assess the patient for any overt behaviors that suggest the patient is ready to talk about anger management. The nurse will also look for signs that the patient is not ready, such as denial of angry feelings. She will also watch for potential triggers for anger that will need to be addressed when teaching anger management skills.

● Key Nursing Interventions to Increase Anger Management Skills

Make expectations clear. For all patients, the nurse will want to make certain that a clear understanding of staff expectations is provided. These expectations will likely include being respectful of others, telling staff when the individual is feeling that he is escalating toward anger, or coming to staff when she has a conflict with another patient (Lowe, 1992). This is best done when the patient first arrives on the unit and when the patient is not in a state of extreme anger. The nurse can explain that he goes over these expectations with all patients. It is important to remember that while it is the nurse's responsibility to provide the behavioral expectations to the patient, a person in crisis may not remember or be able to follow the guidelines. Regardless of this, it is something that the nurse must do and reinforce with each patient.

Share the nurse's assessment with the patient in real time. If the nurse has been successful in building some rapport with the patient, then sharing some of his observations can be a useful intervention. For example, if the nurse observes the patient engaging in behavior that indicates she is escalating, the nurse can step in and ask the patient if she needs help. It is helpful for the nurse to share with the patient what behavior she observed that prompted the nurse's response. Approaching the patient in a helpful manner and avoiding judgmental statements like "remember how you got yesterday, we don't want a repeat of that …" will help this intervention be more successful. In addition, the nurse will want to remember what the patient has said about preferences for contact. The goal should be to assist the patient and to de-escalate the situation so that the patient will be in a frame of mind to listen to feedback and learn from the nurse's observations.

Provide education about the emotion of anger. Ideally, the patient and the nurse will work together to determine the patient's educational needs. The main topics to include in anger management education are

- the purpose of anger as a basic emotion
- the physiological signs that the patient may experience when angry
- the importance of identifying the patient's unique triggers, experiences, and reactions to anger
- ways to cope with the feeling of anger

First, the nurse will want to provide the patient with education about anger being a normal emotion. The patient should know that the purpose of anger is to alert the individual to a potential threat. Angry feelings will often dissipate naturally over time (Olatunji, Lohr, & Bushman, 2007). Second, the nurse will want to teach the patient that anger is associated with signs of arousal such as facial flushing, increased heart rate, increased respiration, and blood pressure. In addition, the nurse may talk with the patient about the fact that the urge to react is natural but not always helpful. The patient may feel the need to run, yell, or hit something; his hands may shake; he may feel shaky and agitated; or he may feel more anxious.

When considering how to teach anger management skills, useful resources are *"Anger Management for Substance Abuse and Mental Health Clients: Participant Workbook"* and *"Anger Management for Substance Abuse and Mental Health Clients: A Cognitive Behavioral Therapy Manual."* These publications can be downloaded or ordered at no charge from the SAMHSA Web site (www.samhsa.gov). Some of the contents can be shared in a group setting or referenced to create a group that fits the patient's needs. Depending on the organization, a staff nurse may be able to conduct a psychoeducational group about anger or advocate for a group led by another team member.

Finally, the nurse may want to educate the patient about "venting." Physical or verbal venting of anger is commonly accepted as a good coping strategy. However, research has demonstrated that verbally or physically "acting out" angry feelings is *not* helpful in improving coping or reducing aggression associated with anger. In fact, ranting endlessly about angry feelings or hitting pillows and tearing up papers is associated with increased risk of future aggressive behaviors (Olatunji et al., 2007).

Teach functional analysis. In order to teach the patient to identify unique triggers, expressions, and reactions to anger, the nurse may use functional analysis. Functional analysis is a technique taken from cognitive behavioral therapy (CBT), which is a therapy that has demonstrated efficacy in treating anger problems (Haddock et al., 2009; Novaco, 1977) (Figure 1.1). There are many resources describing CBT techniques on the SAMSHA website (www.samsha.gov). The website also offers free publications such as *"The TIPS*

Trigger	How did you feel?	What were you thinking?	What did you do?	Positive results	Negative results	Alternative strategies

FIGURE 1.1 Sample Format for a Functional Analysis.

Series: Quick Guide for Clinicians, Brief Interventions and Brief Therapies for Substance Abuse." The process of functional analysis is described in this and other publications.

For the brief inpatient stay, functional analysis provides a structure to help the patient begin to think about how her thoughts and feelings are connected and how they can influence behavior. The nurse can introduce it to a patient as a way to examine her own triggers and angry responses, and to consider alternative responses. Functional analysis can be taught either as part of a group or individually. Regardless of the setting in which it is taught, it is important to teach this as a skill that the patient can learn to do on her own, rather than simply doing it once with a clinician.

Basic functional analysis can be done in a chart form, listing the components to be examined, which include triggers to anger, feelings, thoughts, behaviors, and consequences of behaviors. Patients are instructed to consider a specific instance of anger. Then, the nurse can ask the patient to identify triggers. Triggers can be an internal experience (such as a feeling) or an external experience (such as an interaction). The patient next identifies feelings, physical sensations, thoughts, and behaviors associated with the anger. Next, the patient identifies positive and negative consequences of her actions. Finally, with or without help, the patient reflects on the whole event and identifies any alternative behaviors or coping strategies. The nurse can assist the patient with any part of this analysis. If the patient is having trouble completing the functional analysis, the nurse can use her own observations of the patient and general knowledge about anger to provide suggestions for what he might have been feeling or thinking; the nurse then asks the patient to decide if that applies to this particular patient in the chosen situation.

Offer coping skills. The nurse can offer the patient several active coping skills that have been demonstrated to help angry individuals reduce their arousal from the angry emotion and allow anger to dissipate naturally. These are relaxation techniques such as deep breathing counting to 10, taking a time out or removing oneself from the situation, using distraction or engaging in a soothing, relaxing, or enjoyable activity (see Chapter 13, "Relaxation Techniques," and Chapter 14, "Sensory Interventions"). This last suggestion employs the strategy of having the individual do something that will generate a feeling different from anger (Olatunji et al., 2007). The nurse can help the patient identify what strategies she is willing to try and how she can practice or use these skills on the inpatient unit.

TREATMENT ENGAGEMENT

● Subgoal: Increase Engagement in Treatment

Assessment of Patient's Ability to Engage in Treatment

The assessment of the patient's ability to engage in treatment is similar to the assessment of the patient's readiness to learn anger management skills. Patients who are not cognitively able to participate and unwilling to examine their behavior will not be able to engage completely.

The nurse will want to assess barriers to engagement. Barriers to engaging the patient in treatment are related to the patient's degree of insight, cognitive capacity for insight, and level of readiness for behavioral change.

Intoxicated patients, patients who are psychotic or manic, and patients with severe depression or brain injury will likely not benefit from traditional anger management interventions (Thomas, 2001). In addition, individuals with severe personality disturbance who do not experience any distress about their behavior or who hold certain beliefs about anger, such as "anger is always justified," "catharsis is good," or "I have to express anger whenever I feel it," may also not engage in treatment for anger (Dunbar, 2004; Howells & Day, 2003).

● Key Nursing Interventions to Build Trust and Rapport and Increase Engagement

Although there are patients who have barriers to engagement, there are a few interventions that can help minimize aggression and facilitate patient engagement.

Show respect at all times. In order to build trust and rapport with the patient, it is important for the nurse to spend some time with the patient expressing understanding and concern. One very important point to remember is that civility and courtesy are immensely helpful when someone is angry. The nurse should not "speak down" to the patient, dismiss his feelings and concerns, or present rigid rule enforcement. Consider the example of a patient who is leaning over the nurse's desk or seems to be trying to get to something from behind the nurse's station. The nurse should not respond by saying "You can't go back there," or "Move away from the desk." These remarks will likely trigger an angry response from an individual who may feel that he is being treated as a child. The nurse could instead say, "Do you need something? Can I help you get something?"

Acknowledge and validate the patient's feelings. The nurse will want to acknowledge and validate the anger and any other feelings the patient may be experiencing, such as fear, hurt, or shame. The nurse may also acknowledge real slights or omissions and apologize if it is necessary. The nurse will want to acknowledge any powerlessness the patient may feel or any feelings of perceived threat. Even if the nurse does not agree with what a patient is saying, the nurse can identify and validate the underlying feeling: for example, "It seems like you are feeling unfairly treated and that makes you angry."

PREPARATION FOR DISCHARGE

For all patients, discharge planning should include education regarding medication, primary diagnosis, symptom recognition, and symptom management. For individuals who have benefited from functional analysis or anger management groups during the hospital stay, the nurse and treatment team can discuss a referral to anger management groups on an outpatient basis. Alternatively, the nurse can assist the patient in creating a plan to help cope with any external situations that the patient believes may trigger anger.

TABLE 1.1
Goals, Areas of Assessment, and Interventions for a Patient with Anger

Goal	Assessment	Intervention
Safety		
Prevent or reduce risk for harm to others	Assess history of anger and aggression Consider whether anger is an acute or chronic problem Inquire about patient preferences for and ability to participate in de-escalation Observe the patients behavior, level of physical arousal, and responses to triggers on the unit Use standardized assessment instruments such as the Broset Violence Checklist	Have a plan for preventing aggression Manage environmental triggers Help the patient to de-escalate when needed
Stabilization		
Increase anger management skills	Assess readiness to learn and practice anger management skills Watch for denial that anger is a problem Identify specific triggers	Make expectations clear Share the nurse's assessment with a patient in real time Provide education about the emotion of anger Teach functional analysis Offer coping skills
Treatment Engagement		
Increase engagement in treatment	Assess barriers to treatment engagement: insight, cognitive capacity, and readiness for change	Show respect at all times Acknowledge and validate the patient's feelings

REFERENCES

Abderhalden, C., Needham, I., Miserez, B., Almvik, R., Dassen T., Haug H. J., & Fischer, J. E. (2004). Predicting inpatient violence in acute psychiatric wards using the Broset-violence checklist: A multicentre prospective cohort study. *Journal of Psychiatric and Mental Health Nursing, 11,* 422–427.

Almvik, R., & Woods, P. (1999). Predicting inpatient violence using the Broset violence checklist (BVC). *The International Journal of Psychiatric Nursing Research, 4(3),* 498–504.

Almvik, R., Woods, P., & Rasmussen, K. (2000). The Broset violence checklist: Sensitivity, specificity, and interrater reliability. *Journal of Interpersonal Violence, 15(12),* 1284–1296.

Cheung, R. Y., & Park, J. K. (2010). Anger suppression, interdependent self-control and depression among Asian American and European American college students. *Cultural Diversity and Ethnic Minority Psychology, 16(4),* 517–525.

Davila, Y.R.(1999), Women and Anger. *Journal of Psychosocial Nursing and mental health Services, 37(7),* 25–29.

Dunbar, B. (2004). Anger management: A holistic approach. *Journal of the American Psychiatric Nurses Association, 10(1),* 16–23.

Fischer, A. H., Mosquera, R. M. R., van Vianen, A. E. M., & Manstead, A. S. R. (2004). Gender and culture differences in emotion. *Emotion, 4(1),* 87–94.

Haddock, G., Barrowclough, C., Shaw, J., Dunn, G., Novaco, R. W., & Tarrier, N. (2009). Cognitive-behavioral therapy v. social activity for people with psychosis and a history of violence: Randomized controlled trial. *The British Journal of Psychiatry, 194,* 152–157.

Hollinworth, H., Clark, C., Harland, R., Johnson, L., & Partington, G. (2005). Understanding the arousal of anger: A patient centered approach. *Nursing Standard, 9(37),* 41–47.

Howells, K., & Day, A. (2003). Readiness for anger management: Clinical and theoretical issues. *Clinical Psychology Review, 23,* 319–337.

Johnson, M. E., & Hauser, P. M. (2001). The practices of expert psychiatric nurses: Accompanying the patient to a calmer personal space. *Issues In Mental Health Nursing, 22,* 651–668.

Lowe, T. (1992). Characteristics of effective nursing interventions in the management of challenging behavior. *Journal of Advanced Nursing, 17,* 1226–1232.

Min, S. L., & Suh, S. (2010). The anger syndrome hwa-byung and its comorbidity. *Journal of Affective Disorders, 124,* 211–214.

Murphy, L., & Carsen, V. B. (2010). Anger, aggression and violence. In E. M. Varacolis & M. J. Halter (Eds.), *Foundations of psychiatric mental health nursing: A clinical approach* (6th ed., pp. 565–583). St. Louis, MO: Saunders Elsevier.

Novaco, R. W. (1976). The functions and regulation of the arousal of anger. *American Journal of Psychiatry, 133*(10), 1124–1128.

Novaco, R. W. (1977). Stress inoculation: A cognitive therapy for anger and its application to a case of depression. *Journal of Consulting and Clinical Psychology, 45*(4), 600–608.

Novaco, R. W. (2007). Anger dysregulation. In T. A. Cavall & K. T. Malcolm (Eds.), *Anger, aggression and interventions for interpersonal violence* (pp. 3–54). Hillsdale, NJ: Lawrence Erlbaum.

Olatunji, B. O., Lohr, J. M., & Bushman, B. J. (2007). The pseudo-psychology of venting. In T. A. Cavall & K. T. Malcolm (Eds.), *Anger, aggression and interventions for interpersonal violence* (pp. 119–141). Hillsdale, NJ: Lawrence Erlbaum Associates.

Perry, B. D., & Szalavitz, M. (2006). *The boy who was raised as a dog and other stories from a child psychiatrist notebook.* New York: Basic Books.

Quanbeck, C.D., Mcdermott, B.E. (2008). Inpatient settings. In Simon, R.I. & Tandiff, K., (Eds.), *Textbook of violence assessment and management* (pp. 259–276). Arlington, VA: American Psychiatric Publishing.

Safdar, S., Friedlmeier, W., Matsumoto, D., Kwantes, C. T., Yoo, S. H., & Kakai, H. (2009). Variations of emotional display rules within and across cultures: A comparison between Canada, USA and Japan. *Canadian Journal of Behavioral Science, 41*(1), 1–10.

Substance Abuse and Mental Health Services Administration [SAMHSA]. Retrieved March 10, 2011, from http://www.samhsa.gov

Tangney, J. P., Wagner, P., Fletcher, C., & Gramzow, R. (1992). Shamed into anger? The relation of shame and guilt to anger and self reported aggression. *Journal of Personality and Social Psychology, 62*(4), 669–675.

Thomas, S. P. (2001). Teaching healthy anger management. *Perspectives in Psychiatric Care, 37*(2), 41–47.

Woods, P., Ashley, C., Kayto, D., & Heusdens, C. (2008). Piloting violence and incident reporting measures on one acute mental health inpatient unit. *Issues in Mental Health Nursing, 29*, 455–469.

The Patient With Anxiety

2

Debora Heidtman, Nicole Flanagan,
Debra Spellman, Christopher Paiva,
and Lisa A. Uebelacker

BACKGROUND AND DESCRIPTION

Anxiety is a nonspecific feeling of apprehension or impending doom, which is accompanied by some sort of autonomic response. Anxiety can range from mild to moderate to severe to a state of panic. A mild level of anxiety is considered normal and part of day-to-day living. Feelings of worry or fear before challenging or life-changing events such as starting a new job, buying a house, or going to a job interview are easily justified and considered normal. Anxiety is a useful emotion when it motivates a person to protect himself or his family in times of danger. Mild anxiety is useful when it motivates a student to study for a test or a person to prepare for a job interview. Anxiety is considered a problem when it affects one's ability to perform activities of daily living, interferes with relationships, causes significant distress, or interferes with sleep. Severe anxiety or panic is extremely distressing to a patient.

Some patients may experience *panic attacks*. These are characterized by a sudden onset of intense fear, lasting 1 to 30 minutes. These episodes can be accompanied by intense physical symptoms (see Physical Experience section) and fear of dying, fear of losing control, or a feeling of depersonalization. The person having a panic attack for the first time may not identify the experience as being related to anxiety and may in fact believe she is dying of a serious medical event such as cardiac or respiratory arrest. Because the symptoms of a panic attack and a cardiac event can mimic each other, careful assessment of the physical symptoms is warranted. The patient may be unable to focus and may be so desperate to relieve her anxiety that she strikes out or injures herself. These episodes may seem unprovoked or have an identified trigger. When examined carefully, seemingly unprovoked panic attacks can often be attributed to an intensely fearful reaction to a common somatic symptom (such as an elevated heart rate) that very quickly escalates into a full-blown panic attack (Barlow, 2002).

Behavior

A patient experiencing anxiety may demonstrate it in a variety of ways within the spectrum of anxiety severity. First, the anxious patient may demonstrate *psychomotor agitation.* A mildly anxious patient may demonstrate only foot tapping or leg shaking, whereas the patient with severe anxiety or with a panic attack may pace, rock, or bang his head. Second, a patient may express anxiety by *crying or talking loudly.* A mildly or moderately anxious patient may sit on the unit or be withdrawn in his room and be quietly tearful. In contrast, the severely anxious or panicked patient may be loudly crying or yelling. Third, the nurse can also observe anxiety through the patient's *facial expressions*, which may include grimacing in a mildly anxious patient or a wide-eyed panicked expression in the severely anxious patient.

While on an inpatient unit, the patient with anxiety may be unable to tolerate a lot of stimuli, including other patients who may be loud or agitated, day-to-day noise of an inpatient unit, or noise and activity in the event of medical or psychiatric emergencies. During these times, the anxious patient may retreat or become agitated.

Anxiety affects social interactions. A highly anxious patient may be impulsive and have a low tolerance to wait for his needs to be met. As a result, he may be unable to wait in line for meals or for medication delivery. He may disrupt others by insisting on being first or speaking out of turn. Depending on his level of anxiety, he may be unable to engage with other patients within the milieu. In contrast, an anxious patient may approach staff or other patients seeking reassurance. Those with mild anxiety may seek intermittent reassurance, whereas the highly anxious patient may seek continuous reassurance.

Avoidance is a key behavioral feature of anxiety for many individuals. That is, a person may attempt to avoid whatever makes her anxious, whether it be physiologic sensations in her body, germs or contamination, leaving her room, going to groups, or other social interactions.

Research has revealed that patients with anxiety consistently demonstrate difficulty falling asleep, disrupted sleep with frequent awakenings, and reduced sleep time (Bourdet & Goldenberg, 1994). During evening or night hours, the anxious patient may be awake in common areas, seek staff for reassurance or medication, appear restless in his bed, or call out in his sleep due to nightmares or panic attacks.

Finally, there are some patients who feel very anxious but do not demonstrate it in an expected fashion because they cannot identify their internal experience of distress as being related to anxiety. These patients may respond to unrelated events in an urgent or defensive manner, causing interpersonal conflicts, angry outbursts, and perhaps even "manic" or frantic activity.

Physical Experience

An anxious patient may experience a "flight or fight" response. This involves an increase in adrenaline, which in turn can cause physiological symptoms affecting many systems of the body. Systems affected include

- Cardiac, with resultant symptoms of chest pain, palpitations, hypertension, and elevated heart rate

- Respiratory, with shortness of breath and hyperventilation. Hyperventilation can cause respiratory alkalosis as a result of loss of carbon dioxide (Lambert-Drwiega, 2010)
- Gastrointestinal, with abdominal pain, diarrhea, nausea, or difficulty swallowing
- Genitourinary, with frequent urination
- Integumentary, with pale skin tone or flushing of the skin, or diaphoresis
- Neurological, with symptoms such as blurred vision, tunnel vision, dilated pupils, tremor, tingling of the extremities, headache, dizziness or faintness, or sleep disturbance

The physical experience may mirror the level of anxiety the patient experiences. For example, a patient with mild anxiety may report a few mild physical symptoms, such as shortness of breath. In contrast, a severely anxious patient or a patient having a panic attack may experience many severe symptoms all at once.

Cognition

The patient's anxiety is often based on the perception of threat or loss. The patient's ability to verbally express the source of her fear can vary widely from patient to patient. Some patients may not be able to express that they are anxious or why they are anxious. Some may deny anxiety all together. In contrast, some may clearly be able to state that they are experiencing anxiety and even identify a trigger to their feelings. Some patients may express fear of how they will handle major life events, such as a divorce or a loss of home. Other patients may express anxiety about seemingly smaller problems, for example, missing a physician's appointment, and fearing that she will be terminated as a patient. The degree of anxiety may seem out of proportion to the feared event; however, it is important to remember that this experience is potentially very intense for the patient and the nurse should take it seriously.

Some anxious patients may describe a feeling of impending doom. They may ruminate about their fears or have seemingly irrational beliefs that interfere with daily functioning. They may describe their thoughts as "racing." Depending on the severity of the anxiety, they may have difficulty thinking about or focusing on topics unrelated to their anxiety. The feelings may incapacitate the patient such that they view suicide or self-harm as an option to reduce or relieve their anxiety.

Affect

Anxiety is a fundamental human emotion. Words that may be used to describe varying degrees or types of anxiety include worried, apprehensive, nervous, unsettled, scared, or terrified. Patients may say they are "on edge," "freaking out," or "crawling out of my skin." The anxious person may also be irritable or guarded in reaction to the experience of anxiety, or may appear sad or withdrawn due to anxiety or hopelessness about having such severe anxiety.

Context

Anxiety is common among psychiatric inpatients. Anxiety can be present in a spectrum of psychiatric disorders. "Anxiety disorders" include generalized anxiety disorder, panic disorder, posttraumatic stress disorder, obsessive–compulsive disorder, social anxiety disorder, and specific phobias (American Psychiatric Association, 2000).

Anxiety disorders may be differentiated by the types of fears and behaviors that a person has. When a person has seemingly unprovoked panic attacks, persistent concerns about having additional attacks, and/or fear of losing control or "going crazy," she may have panic disorder.

A patient who has experienced a panic attack in the past may be so fearful about its reoccurrence that she becomes isolative and avoids leaving the house (or participating in the milieu). This is called "agoraphobia." Generalized anxiety disorder is characterized by pervasive worry about many domains of life. Posttraumatic stress disorder is considered an anxiety disorder because the individuals with this disorder are fearful of thoughts, feelings, events, or places that remind them of a trauma. Obsessive–compulsive disorder can involve fear of what will occur if one has certain types of thoughts and/or when certain cognitive or behavioral rituals are not performed. Finally, social anxiety disorder can be characterized by fear of very specific social situations (such as speaking in public, eating in public, or using public bathrooms) or can be generalized to many different social situations and interactions.

Anxiety can also be a prominent feature of mood disorders, including unipolar major depression and bipolar disorder. The frequency of co-occurring psychiatric disorders and substance abuse is high in patients with anxiety; for example, one study reported that 90% of patients with generalized anxiety disorder have another psychiatric disorder (Woodman, 1997).

The prevalence of medical disorders such as cardiovascular disease or gastroesophageal reflux disease is higher in patients with anxiety disorders than in those without anxiety disorders (Mizyed, Fass, & Fass, 2009; Olafiranye, Jean-Louis, Zizi, Nunes, & Vincent, 2011). Patients with anxiety disorders also have an increased risk of myocardial infarction (Scherrer et al., 2010). Many medical issues can also lead to a patient experiencing anxiety. One example is a patient with pulmonary disease who experiences anxiety in the context of fear of being unable to breath. In addition, diseases such as hypothyroidism can create a feeling of anxiety or panic. Some medications such as bronchodilators have a stimulant effect that may contribute to symptoms of anxiety. The feeling of anxiety can also result from withdrawal of medications such as antidepressants or substances such as benzodiazepines or alcohol.

Ataque de nervios is an idiom of distress seen in Latino cultures (American Psychiatric Association, 2000). Common symptoms of *ataques de nervios* include "uncontrollable shouting, attacks of crying, trembling, heat in the chest rising into the head, and verbal or physical aggression" (American Psychiatric Association, 2000, p. 899). There is usually a sense of being out of control. There are other less common symptoms as well, such as dissociative experiences. *Ataques* bear some similarities to a panic attack but most *ataques* occur following a precipitating event. Individuals who report *ataques de nervios* are more likely to meet criteria for mood, anxiety, and substance-use disorders than those who do not have *ataques de nervios* (Guarnaccia et al., 2010). These individuals are also likely to experience fear of the physiological sensations of arousal, that is, they experience fear when they note that their heart is beating quickly, they feel tingling, or feel other bodily sensations (Hinton, Chong, Pollack, Barlow, & McNally, 2008).

POTENTIAL BARRIERS TO BEING THERAPEUTIC

The nurse is challenged in several ways by the anxious patient. A patient's anxiety and frequent need for reassurance may create a feeling of anxiety or be overwhelming for the nurse. The nurse may give medications or treatment that may not be indicated to relieve the nurse's own anxiety or to appease the patient. Conversely, patients who express medical concerns or fears that the nurse may feel are trite or invalid may be discounted by the nurse. The nurse will need to consistently return to interventions, described below, that show respect for the patient and his experience.

OVERVIEW OF NURSING CARE GOALS

1. Safety
   - Prevent or reduce risk of harm to self
   - Maintain patient's physiological functioning within normal limits
2. Stabilization
   - Help to reduce symptoms of anxiety and agitation
3. Engagement
   - Assist patients with engaging in treatment on the unit

SAFETY

● **Subgoal: Prevent or Reduce Risk of Harm to Self**

The experience of anxiety or the inability to relieve anxiety may be so distressing to a patient that he may escalate to self-harm. The diagnosis of patients with an anxiety disorder is strongly associated with suicide attempts (Boden, Fergusson, & Horwood 2007). For comprehensive treatment of assessment and prevention of risk for self-harm, please see Chapter 5, "The Patient With Nonsuicidal Self-Injury," and Chapter 9, "The Patient Who Is Suicidal." Here, we focus only on issues specifically related to anxiety and suicide.

Assessment of Risk for Harm to Self

In report. When the nurse hears or suspects that a patient may be very anxious, it is critical that she learns about the risk for self-harm, including important risk factors such as patient's history of self-harm, as well as whether intense anxiety has played a role in self-harm behaviors in the past.

Next, the nurse will want to know about acute triggers for increased anxiety, as these may be the times when the patient is most likely to harm himself. Finally, the nurse will enquire about previous strategies used to avoid self-injurious behavior. These strategies may be the same strategies used to calm the patient when he is particularly anxious, or to prevent the onset of panic attacks or extreme anxiety.

One-to-one contact. Although self-harm is not the only thing that the nurse will want to assess during this contact, it should be a priority. The nurse could say, "Have you been feeling anxious today?" If the patient responds affirmatively, the nurse will then explore thoughts of self-harm by asking, "Are these feelings so distressing that you have thoughts of hurting yourself?" If the patient acknowledges these types of thoughts, the nurse may then enquire about a plan, risk factors, and protective factors.

On the unit. Some anxiety-related cues that might indicate that the patient is at risk for self-injury or a suicide attempt include

- Increased behavioral signs of agitation or anxiety, such as inability to maintain eye contact, restlessness, or pacing
- Statements like "I cannot take it any more" or "I can't do this anymore"

● **Key Nursing Interventions to Prevent Risk of Harm to Self**

Be proactive when an anxiety trigger is anticipated or has just occurred. This is when the nurse will be particularly vigilant about looking for evidence of self-harm or thoughts of self-harm. Assertively treating the patient's anxiety and agitation, as described below, should reduce the risk of self-harm.

● Subgoal: Maintain Patient's Physiological Functioning Within Normal Limits

As mentioned earlier, the experience of anxiety can affect many systems of the body and lead to medical instability, which in turn can lead to a major medical problem such as hypertension and then a cerebrovascular event. Poor fluid intake can lead to orthostasis and electrolyte imbalance, which in turn can lead to increased risk for fall or life-threatening cardiac arrhythmias.

Assessment of Impaired Physiological Functioning
In report. Because anxiety affects many systems of the body, the nurse needs to understand what the patient's physiologic functioning was during the previous shift. A patient's prior physical concerns may be an indicator of what to expect during the next shift. Physical concerns to address include

- Elevations in vital signs. The nurse will want to understand the patient's baseline and current values so that variation can be recognized and addressed
- Cardiac issues, including complaints of chest pain. It is important for the nurse to know whether there is a history of pulmonary or cardiac issues, as well as what works to alleviate the chest pain
- Gastrointestinal distress, including pain, nausea, or dry mouth. Increased levels of adrenaline (part of the flight or fight response) can result in increased acidity in stomach content and gastrointestinal bleeding. The nurse will also want to know about food and fluid intake and regularity of elimination to assess for adequate hydration and nutrition
- Pain and neurologic symptoms, including headaches, blurred vision, or dizziness. The nurse will want to know about severity of pain and what has worked to alleviate the pain in the past

The nurse will also want to know what medications the patient has received for anxiety and whether these medications had a positive (or negative) impact on these physiological concerns.

One-to-one contact. A good time for the nurse to assess physiologic concerns with the patient is during the assessment of vital signs. The nurse should provide privacy so that the patient can discuss his physical symptoms without fear of embarrassment. In the context of asking general questions about the patient's overall well being, such as how he is feeling, the nurse can ask about appetite, food intake, and elimination patterns. The nurse will also ask about pain or discomfort. However, she will do so in a general way so as to avoid leading the patient to endorse somatic symptoms he may not be experiencing. For example, the nurse might say, "Tell me what your day has been like so far," or ask, "How are you feeling?" Unless already established as an ongoing problem, she would tend not to ask, "Are you having any chest pain?" The nurse will also observe behavior to evaluate if the behavior matches the reported symptoms. However, she should keep in mind that the expression of pain and physical distress can vary widely from patient to patient. For example, one patient may sit quietly when experiencing pain while another may be more demonstrative and talk about pain and physical symptoms in different parts of the body. Because pain and other physical symptoms such as nausea are so subjective, it is impossible for the nurse to know what the patient is "truly" feeling, and she must strive to take the patient's report at face value and understand that the patient truly is suffering.

If the patient reports chest pain, the nurse must always assess it further and not assume it is an anxiety symptom (although it may well be). If chest pain is mild, the nurse will elicit information about the pain, including severity, location, and type. She can ask the patient to describe the pain in his own words. She can also ask if there was a precipitant to the pain, if it has occurred previously, and what has helped in the past. She will take care to appear calm and confident and take the patient's vital signs. If vital signs are normal, chest pain should be communicated to the patient's physician in a timely manner and monitored until recommendations are made. If there are irregularities in vital signs, including pulse, blood pressure, respiration, and oxygen saturation, the nurse should take immediate action to have the chest pain evaluated further.

On the unit. The nurse will evaluate the patient's nutritional status. He will note whether she initiates getting food at mealtimes or she needs to be prompted to eat, will note how much of the meal is eaten, and will always be on the lookout for any observable indications of distress or physical pain through facial expressions or modification in bodily movements.

● Key Nursing Interventions to Maintain Patient's Physiological Functioning Within Normal Limits

Treat elevated vital signs. The nurse will review the patient's vital signs to determine whether they fall within normal parameters for the patient. In particular, anxious patients may have an elevated heart rate, blood pressure, or respiration. If vital signs are abnormal, the nurse will want to evaluate available medication that can be administered to regulate vital signs. As the nurse administers the medications, he can review concerns that the patient might have and provide support and education about the physiological symptoms and their treatment. He will want to make sure that the patient knows she will be monitored frequently, which may be reassuring to the patient. If vital signs show a mild to moderate elevation from the patient's baseline, the nurse will reassess as determined by the parameters of the institution or the physician. If there is no relief from medications, the nurse will want to consult with the patient's physician.

If the elevation in vital signs is severe, the nurse should provide constant monitoring and a calming environment with low-lighting and quiet or soothing music. Information and instructions to the patient should be brief, as the patient may not process the content of lengthy conversations or extensive information. The nurse will notify the physician immediately.

Provide for fluid and nutritional needs. If the patient has a dry mouth or low fluid intake, has missed a meal, or is not eating, the nurse can take some actions to encourage fluid and nutrition intake. The nurse should let the patient know what the menu choices are and ask them what they would prefer. If the patient is not interested in the choices, the nurse may consider discussing food preferences with the patient and working with the dietary department so as to provide desired foods. Sometimes small but frequent meals will be more palatable than larger, less frequent meals. She may also see if family members can bring in foods from home that might be soothing to the patient. The nurse may discuss with the treatment team the need for a nutrition consult.

Provide support and assistance if a patient is hyperventilating. During episodes of hyperventilation, the nurse will ensure privacy and a quiet area when possible. However, in the midst of a panic attack, a patient may be unable to respond to suggestions to move to a different location. In those times, the nurse may provide privacy by asking other patients to kindly leave the area. When the patient is hyperventilating, the nurse can provide direct eye contact, firm direction, and model slow deep breathing until the experience passes. Throughout, she can reassure the patient that the episode will, by necessity, be time limited and that she will stay with the patient until it subsides.

She may also consider other sensory interventions. Please see Chapter 14 "Sensory Interventions."

STABILIZATION

● Subgoal: Help to Reduce Symptoms of Anxiety and Agitation

Assessment of Anxiety and Agitation

In report. The nurse will want to know about the patient's general level of agitation and anxiety on the previous shift (i.e., mild, moderate, or severe), as well as any episodes of acute anxiety (i.e., panic attacks). Was the patient able to attend and participate in groups? If not, why? Was it due to anxiety? It is useful to know which specific behavioral, physiological, and cognitive symptoms each patient tends to experience and if any specific anxiety triggers have been identified for that patient. The nurse will also ask about effective strategies for managing anxiety. Were medications needed on the previous shift or offered by staff? If so, did they work? Did the patient use any sensory modalities, and what was the effectiveness? The nurse should also note what medications the patient is taking to determine whether any of these could be a contributor to anxiety.

One-to-one contact. With an anxious patient, the nurse should introduce herself as the contact person as soon as possible in the shift and tell the patient that he can come to her if he has a problem or issue. The anxious patient should know ahead of time that the nurse will be meeting with him for a one-to-one contact, the purpose of the meeting, and the approximate time and the length of the meeting. This may help to reduce anxiety. The nurse should let the patient know that if, for some reason, she is unable to meet with the patient at that time, she or someone else will inform the patient as soon as possible.

The patient's ability to tolerate contact will vary depending on the level of anxiety and how the treatment course is progressing. During times of severe anxiety, he may be unable to tolerate this type of contact. When the time comes for the one-to-one contact, the nurse will ask the patient if this is a good time to talk and allow the patient opportunity to defer the meeting until she feels ready. If the patient is ready, the nurse should provide a low stimuli area for the conversation. Note that this contact may be conducted in ways other than sitting down and talking face-to-face, for example, during assessment of vital signs or by walking with the patient as she paces on the unit.

The nurse will proceed with the conversation in an unhurried manner and begin by asking if there are any specific concerns that the nurse can assist the patient with and how he is feeling in general. Next, the nurse may assess current and recent levels of anxiety. For example, she may say, "Tell me what your anxiety level is like today. How is it different from previous days?" The nurse can also look for physical cues to determine whether the patient's response is congruent with his observed behaviors. If the patient's behaviors do not appear to correspond to what he is saying, the nurse may enquire. For example, she could say, "You have told me that you are not anxious, but I see that you are fidgeting and moving around a lot. I wonder if you are uncomfortable or having any thoughts you would like to share" She could also provide the patient with a comparison of a time she had observed him in a calmer state: "I saw earlier that you were sitting in a group and participating. How you were feeling at that time? How is that different from now?"

If the patient identifies times of increased anxiety, the nurse may ask about triggers: "Does anxiety increase when thinking about anything in particular?" or "Are you able to identify what upsets you or causes you anxiety?" If the nurse has observed what she believes to be certain triggers, she may offer these possibilities to the patient to see if he has identified the same triggers.

The nurse will ask about response to treatment. Questions could include: "Did you go to any groups today? How was that for you?" "Do you feel like treatment is helping your anxiety?" "Are you feeling better than on admission—if so, why do you think that is?" "Do you feel your medication is helping your anxiety?" "What have you found to be helpful with anxiety in the past?"

Because this patient is known to be anxious, the nurse should watch for the patient's ability to tolerate the conversation during the interaction. Cues that he may be unable to continue the conversation can include body movement such as foot tapping or eye movements such as darting eyes or poor eye contact. If the nurse notices this, she may say, "It seems like you may have had enough talking for now—is that right?" If the patient agrees, the nurse will end the interaction.

On the unit. The nurse can also assess level of anxiety or agitation by watching the patient's behavior on the unit. Indicators of lower anxiety include calm interactions with others, ability to sit in a chair, ability to respond appropriately to staff or patients, use of sensory items or other coping strategies, ability to seek out staff when he needs something rather than isolating or escalating, and ability to participate in milieu and group treatments. Indicators of higher levels of anxiety include pacing, fidgeting, loud or pressured speech, irritability, impulsiveness, isolation, intrusiveness, and hypersensitivity to noise of others or the unit.

The nurse will also want to assess whether other patients can tolerate the anxious patient's behavior if he is loud, pacing, or otherwise potentially disruptive. The nurse needs to consider the risk of others becoming agitated in response to the anxious patient's behavior.

● **Key Nursing Interventions for Reducing Anxiety or Agitation**

Provide a calm environment and structure to the patient's day. The nurse should provide for an environment that is the least stimulating as possible. Ways to achieve this may include bringing the patient to a quieter area of the unit, decreasing the lighting on the unit, or allowing the patient to be in the quiet area of his room or in a sensory room as needed. Related to this, the nurse may want to try to ensure that the patient's roommate is not intrusive, loud, psychotic, or overly talkative.

The nurse may assist the patient to develop a written plan for activities each shift. This should include group times, relaxation times, exercise times, and meal times. When developing the plan, the nurse should help identify and make available calming activities, such as journaling or sensory interventions. The nurse can encourage the patient to carry this "structured schedule" with her and refer to it as frequently as needed. This schedule will create a rhythm to the day, minimize uncertainty, and ensure adequate periods of rest and relaxation.

Provide education about anxiety symptoms. The nurse can help the patient to identify symptoms of anxiety and to better understand what he is experiencing. The nurse can describe anxiety as a normal human emotion that actually serves an adaptive function. That is, it is the body's way of preparing to either fight or flee because of danger. The problem, for this particular patient, may be that this normal system is very sensitive or responds to events that may not actually put her in danger.

Further, patients who experience panic attacks should understand that the experience is time limited and generally lasts no more than 10 minutes. Although panic attacks are emotionally debilitating, it is critical that the patient understands panic attacks are not life threatening and the patient is not "going crazy."

Identify times or triggers for high stress and anxiety and be proactive. Examples of times or activities that might trigger higher levels of anxiety include visiting hours; loud activities, including watching television; unstructured time; or time in large groups of people. The nurse should work with the patient to identify individualized times or triggers for higher anxiety. The nurse can suggest that the patient use journaling as a way to identify potential triggers to these events. That is, when the patient is feeling anxious or after having a panic attack, the patient can write about what he was doing, thinking, and feeling just before the anxiety began. Doing this repeatedly may help the patient to discover patterns.

Once triggers are identified, the nurse can work with the patient to design a proactive plan for how the patient can manage these times or triggers. This plan can include the following elements:

- The nurse checks in with the patient to see how he is doing and assesses his comfort level. The patient can also come up to the nurse to let her know that he thinks his anxiety is increasing.
- The nurse offers diversional activities, relaxation strategies, prn medications, or a change in environment, such as the sensory room.
- The nurse may offer one-to-one contact or brief but frequent contacts during this time.

Knowing that there is a plan to handle difficult situations may be comforting to the anxious patient.

Teach or encourage ways to relax. The nurse can teach the patient, or encourage him to use, deep breathing or imagery techniques for relaxation. (Please see Chapter 13, "Relaxation Techniques.") The nurse can also encourage the use of sensory interventions for comfort. (Please see Chapter 14, "Sensory Interventions.")

Provide education on sleep medications and sleep hygiene. The nurse can educate the patient on the importance of sleep as an essential component to well-being.

If the patient is having difficulty sleeping, the nurse can tell the patient about medications that are available to aid sleep. The nurse can talk about the best time to take these medications, that is, close enough to bedtime so that these medications work, but not too late so that the patient will not be sedated when it is time to get up and be active.

In addition to medications, there are other things a patient can do to improve sleep during the hospital stay and beyond. These include

- Going to bed at the same time and waking up at the same time regardless of sleep quality and quantity in order to get the body on a schedule
- Being sure to engage in exercise daily
- Avoiding strenuous activities, exercise, or heavy meals at least 2 hours before bedtime
- Avoiding any stimulating agents, such as nicotine, caffeine, and even chocolate a few hours before bed
- Limiting the use of alcohol as it will disrupt quality of sleep and leave the patient feeling more tired
- Avoiding daytime napping
- Having a nighttime routine that is relaxing, such as soothing music, a warm bath, or a shower
- Keeping the bedroom cool, dark, and quiet

Provide space to rest if needed. A high level of adrenaline can lead to fatigue following an acute episode of anxiety. Medications administered may also lead to sedation. Therefore, the patient may need to rest following an episode of severe anxiety. The nurse can encourage the patient to find a quiet environment. The patient and nurse may need to evaluate the need for visitors or participation in groups at that time. The nurse can let the patient know that this experience is normal after an episode of severe anxiety and that the patient can opt out of group participation if necessary.

Provide appropriate medication education and collaborate around medication provision. Anxious patients may be anxious about taking medications. Some patients may be fearful about taking new medications or generic medications. Others may be very worried about side effects. If this is the case, medication education may be particularly helpful. The nurse will collaborate with the patient and educate him about the indication or purpose of the medication and how it may help to improve symptoms. Note that the best time for extensive education may *not* be when the patient is extremely anxious, but when he is feeling calmer and is more able to retain the information.

Another way for the nurse to collaborate with the patient is, if the patient is on multiple medications, to assess his ability to take all the medications at once. The nurse may ask how the patient takes the medication at home. The patient might prefer to take the medications over a period of time; often this can be arranged within the policy of the individual organization.

Finally, the nurse should be aware that if a patient has severe anxiety at the time of routine medication administration, it may be best for the nurse to go to the patient rather than expecting the patient to come to him.

Provide appropriate prn medications. The prn medications for anxiety and agitation may include anxiolytics, such as benzodiazepines, or antipsychotics. Some patients may have more than one option. The nurse should be proactive and offer medication prior to a crisis situation whenever possible. That is, when patient is exhibiting signs of escalation or showing behaviors that previously led up to high levels of anxiety, the nurse may want to offer medications. He may speak to the patient, ask how she is feeling, and say that he wondered if a prn medication would be helpful in this particular situation. He may comment that the medication worked for the patient before. He will offer a choice when it is available and may include combinations of prn medications as one may work to potentiate the effect of another.

TREATMENT ENGAGEMENT

● **Subgoal: Assist Patients With Engagement in Treatment on the Unit**

Assessment of Ability to Engage in Treatment

When a person is very anxious, it may be hard for her to focus on the environment or on others; instead, she is focused on anxious thoughts, feelings, and sensations. The following may be indicators of increased ability to engage in treatment:

- Improved eye contact
- Ability to sit for longer periods of time
- Decreased psychomotor agitation
- Increased participation in social or group activities
- Ability to follow through on several-step directions
- Articulation of needs verbally instead of the nurse having to speculate based on nonverbal behavior
- Tendency to start asking questions about treatment
- Increased ability to make decisions for oneself (e.g., about what to eat)
- Increased insight into the relationship between anxiety, one's behavior, and one's environment

● **Key Nursing Interventions to Increase Engagement in Treatment**

Treat the patient calmly, professionally, and respectfully. When a patient is anxious, it is important that the nurse is calm, confident, and supportive and avoids using a loud, rapid, or pressured tone of voice. He should try not to act hurried or display anxiety. He should not catastrophize the patient's symptoms. For example, if the patient is hyperventilating, the nurse should treat this problem calmly. The nurse should not say, "If you keep breathing that fast, something bad may happen," as this could escalate the patient's symptoms or trigger other symptoms.

When discussing anxiety, the nurse should take care to respect and validate the patient's experience. That is, he should not say, "Everything will be fine," or dismiss the patient's thoughts, feelings, and symptoms. If the patient is expressing physical concerns, for example, a racing heart or trouble catching her breath, the nurse might say, "It appears that you are having difficulty," and encourage the patient to take a deep breath and focus on her breathing. The nurse may offer to check her vital signs so as not to discount the patient's reported symptoms. At the same time that he acknowledges the discomfort of the symptoms and checks to make sure the patient is medically safe, the nurse may also educate the patient that her anxiety may cause these physical symptoms.

The nurse may want to adjust the perimeter of the rules to individualize treatment for the patient. The ability to show flexibility will provide a de-escalating and less stressful experience for the patient. For example, if a visitor is unable to come during visiting hours but has a calming effect on the patient, the nurse may allow that visitor to visit outside of those hours.

In order to maintain trust and credibility, the nurse will make sure he follows through on promises. He will not make promises that he cannot follow through on. For example, if a patient is requesting privileges to go outside on pass, the nurse must be honest and let her know that this decision would need to be discussed with her physician. The nurse will not provide false hope.

Finally, the nurse will be sure to familiarize the anxious patient with the unit and milieu. Because she may have difficulty concentrating and remembering things, the nurse may need to repeat this information. For the same reason, the nurse may need to reidentify himself each time he approaches the patient. Doing this in a calm and non-judgmental way may be reassuring to the patient.

Match patients with the appropriate groups. The nurse will assess the ability of the patient to engage in different types of group programming and match the patient's level of ability to engage with the type of group that is taking place. For example, if the patient is very anxious, he may be unable to concentrate in a cognitive behavioral therapy group, but he may be able to participate in a relaxation or exercise group. Social anxiety may also interfere with engagement in group treatments. The nurse can make going to groups less intimidating by saying that the patient can sit near the outskirts and just listen and leave any time. The nurse should approach the anxious patient and encourage him to attend group, but not demand or require it. The nurse can also assist in finding individualized activities if the patient is unable to tolerate group format.

PREPARATION FOR DISCHARGE

It is important for the anxious patient to know ahead of time that he will be discharged on a particular day. On the day of discharge, the nurse will remind the patient of the plan and review the institution's process for discharge. Because there are different elements of aftercare that need to be secured (follow-up appointments, prescriptions, transportation, etc.), frequent updates can be reassuring and informative to the patient. This will help to minimize anxiety and distress common with patients at the time of discharge. The nurse can remind the patient to gather all of his belongings so that when the moment for discharge arrives, he is prepared to leave. When all preparations are completed, the nurse should provide privacy when reviewing the medication and aftercare plan and plan for the fact that the anxious patient may have a lot of questions and need further reassurance.

TABLE 2.1
Goals, Areas of Assessment, and Interventions for a Patient
With Anxiety

Goal	Assessment	Intervention
Safety		
Prevent or reduce risk of harm to self	Know whether there is a history of self-harm behaviors and ask about current self-harm ideation	Be proactive when an anxiety trigger is anticipated or has just occurred
	Understand what triggers severe anxiety in the patient; this may lead to self injurious behaviors	See also Chapter 5, "The Patient With Nonsuicidal Self-Injury," and Chapter 9, "The Patient Who Is Suicidal"
	Monitor for increased behavioral signs of agitation or anxiety	
	See also Chapter 5, "The Patient With Nonsuicidal Self-Injury," and Chapter 9, "The Patient Who Is Suicidal"	
Maintain patient's physiological functioning within normal limits	Understand patient's baseline level of physiological functioning	Treat elevated vital signs
	Assess vital signs	Provide for fluid and nutritional needs
	Assess any concerns about cardiac issues or chest pain, gastrointestinal distress, other pain, or neurological symptoms	Provide support and assistance if a patient is hyperventilating
	Evaluate appetite, food intake, and elimination patterns	

(cont.)

TABLE 2.1
Goals, Areas of Assessment, and Interventions for a Patient
With Anxiety　(*cont.*)

Goal	Assessment	Intervention
Stabilization		
Help to reduce symptoms of anxiety and agitation	Learn about level of anxiety and interventions that helped during previous shift Ask patient about her level of anxiety Identify triggers for anxiety Ask patient about his response to treatment Observe anxious behaviors and agitations on the unit	Provide a calm environment and structure to the patient's day Provide education about anxiety symptoms Identify times or triggers for high stress and anxiety, and be proactive Teach or encourage ways to relax Provide education on sleep medications and sleep hygiene Provide space to rest if needed Provide appropriate medication education and collaborate around medication provision Provide appropriate prn medication
Treatment Engagement		
Assist patients with engagement in treatment on the unit	Observe for indicators of increased ability to engage in treatment	Treat the patient calmly, professionally, and respectfully Match patients with the appropriate groups

REFERENCES

American Psychiatric Association. (2000). *Diagnostic and statistical manual of mental disorders* (4th ed.). Washington, DC: Author.

Barlow, D. H. (2002). *Anxiety and its disorders: The nature and treatment of anxiety and panic* (2nd ed.). New York: The Guilford Press.

Boden, J. M., Fergusson, D. M., & Horwood, L. J. (2007). Anxiety disorders and suicidal behaviours in adolescence and young adulthood: Findings from a longitudinal study. *Psychological Medicine, 37*, 431–440. doi:10.1017/S0033291706009147

Bourdet, C., & Goldenberg, F. (1994). Insomnia in anxiety: Sleep EEG changes. *Journal of Psychosomatic Research, 38*(1), 93–104.

Guarnaccia, P. J., Lewis-Fernandez, R., Pincay, I. M., Shrout, P., Guo, J., Torres, M.,…Alegria, M. (2010). *Ataque de nervios* as a marker of social and psychiatric vulnerability: Results from the NLAAS. *International Journal of Psychiatry, 56*(3), 298–309.

Hinton, D. E., Chong, R., Pollack, M. H., Barlow, D. H., & McNally, R. J. (2008). *Ataque de nervios:* Relationship to anxiety sensitivity and dissociation predisposition. *Depression and Anxiety, 25*, 489–495.

Lambert-Drwiega, A. (May 19, 2010). *Respiratory alkalosis*. Retrieved September 26, 2011, from http://emedicine.medscape.com/article/301680-overview

Mizyed, I., Fass, S. S., & Fass, R. (2009). Gastro-esophageal reflux disease and psychological comorbidity. *Alimentary Pharmacology & Therapeutics, 29*(4), 351–358.

Olafiranye, O., Jean-Louis, G., Zizi, F., Nunes, J., & Vincent, M. T. (2011). Anxiety and cardiovascular risk: Review of epidemiological and clinical evidence. *Mind & Brain, 2*(1), 32–37.

Scherrer, J. F., Chrusciel, T., Zeringue, A., Garfield, L. D., Hauptman, P. J., Lustman, P. J., & True, W. R. (2010). Anxiety disorders increase risk for incident myocardial infarction in depressed sand non-depressed veteran's administration patients. *American Heart Journal, 159*(5), 772–779.

Woodman, C. L. (1997). The natural history of generalized anxiety disorder: A review. *Medscape Psychiatry & Mental Health eJournal, 2*(3). Retrieved October 3, 2011, from http://www.medscape.com/viewarticle/431268

The Patient With Disorganized Behavior

3

Judy L. Sheehan, Idrialis Perez,
and Mary Trainor

BACKGROUND AND DESCRIPTION

Behavior

A disorganized patient is one who behaves in a manner that lacks order, appears illogical, is unpredictable, or otherwise seems to reflect impaired cognitive functioning. Patients who are disorganized may have difficulties with *activities of daily living,* such as bathing, dressing, eating, and toileting, as the patient may be unable to complete the individual steps necessary for these basic tasks. The patient may attempt to dress himself and come out of the room with socks on his feet and a hat on his head but not trousers or shirt. These patients may appear dirty, disheveled, or emaciated.

Patients may also have difficulty with *communication and social behavior.* A disorganized person may be unable to read, write, or understand verbal instructions or directions. This person may have incoherent speech or may not speak much. In addition to verbal language, this person may have trouble interpreting nonverbal behavior and correctly reading social cues. This may lead to violations of social norms, such as wearing inappropriate clothing, eating from other people's plates, or undressing in public. This patient also may demonstrate disinhibition or confusion, and become lost, wander into other patient rooms, disrupt interactions, invade people's personal space, and engage in unprovoked confrontations.

Finally, the patient may engage in *repetitive, purposeless, or nongoal-directed tasks*, such as continually filling a coffee cup even though it is overflowing or standing up and sitting down repeatedly. This patient may pace, pick at unseen items, cry out, or otherwise communicate emotional distress even if it appears that there is no external provocation (Andersson & Bergedalen, 2002; Johnston, 2008; McCabe, Quayle, Beirne, & Duane, 2002; Peters et al., 2008; Smith, 2005).

Cognition

Disorganized behaviors are very often associated with (and perhaps the result of) cognitive impairment. Cognitive impairment is a very broad term that could include fragmented thinking; difficulty with logical thought; impaired attention, concentration, and memory; problems with planning and information processing; and poor judgment. The patient may demonstrate concrete thinking, perseveration, and loss of cognitive flexibility. There is great variability in cognitive abilities and processes. Impairment may range from mild to severe; be limited to specific cognitive domains or be widespread; and be transient, chronic, or fluctuating from hour to hour or day to day.

Affect

The affect of the disorganized person will vary considerably depending upon the situation. Disorganized individuals are frequently anxious and fearful, with marked underlying agitation. This person may seem bewildered, frustrated, irritable, sad, happy, silly, or angry, depending on how the person is interpreting internal or external stimuli. Affect may be labile or fixed, may be appropriate or inappropriate, and may range widely with the correspondence between affect and apparent environmental stimuli getting more tenuous with increasing cognitive impairment.

Context

Disorganized behavior can be associated with any number of psychiatric and medical conditions. Causes may include

- *Delirium*, which can be caused by infection, illness, alcohol, or drugs. Delirium is usually considered to be transient
- *Neurological problems such as dementia or traumatic brain injuries.* Depending upon the severity of damage, these may not be transient but may be chronic and stable, or chronic and worsening
- *Psychiatric disorders such as schizophrenia, bipolar disorder, or other disorders with prominent psychotic symptoms that disrupt rational thought and behavior* (Chowdhury R., 2003). In these cases, disorganized behavior may improve after an acute exacerbation of the disorder is brought under control
- *Long-standing developmental delays.* Disorganized behavior may be chronic in these cases although it may improve with a stable and predictable environment (Johnston, 2008; Lippert-Gruner, 2006; Peters et al., 2008)

Identifying the cause of the disorganization gives the nurse an understanding of prognosis and helps to guide medical treatment and choice of nursing goals.

POTENTIAL BARRIERS TO BEING THERAPEUTIC

Communication with a disorganized person can be very difficult. Whether the patient is distracted by psychosis, limited by cognitive deficits, or unable to communicate due to delirium, the nurses' tools for building and maintaining a therapeutic relationship will be limited. Nurses, who are accustomed to using a verbal approach in interactions with patients, will need to depend more readily on nonverbal communication along with environmental management in order to ensure the well being of all. This will require the nurse to be in the physical vicinity of the patient frequently, often at the expense of other nursing activities such as medication management, communication with other team members, or medical treatments. Repeating instructions and directions for a confused patient, refocusing activity, and redirecting paths of ambulation while also accomplishing the standard nursing actions required on an inpatient unit will challenge the nurse to multitask safely. The nurse may experience frustration and anxiety in the face of conflicting agendas and react with anger and impatience toward the patients.

OVERVIEW OF NURSING CARE GOALS

1. Safety
   - Prevent or reduce self-harm
   - Prevent or reduce confrontations between patient and others
2. Stabilization
   - Decrease disorganized behavior and associated anxiety
3. Engagement
   - Involve patient in unit-based activities to the extent possible

SAFETY

● Subgoal: Prevent or Reduce Self-harm

Depending on the patient's level of disorganization and underlying cognitive impairment, the patient may be at risk for accidental injury through falls or other means.

This person might engage in unsafe and high-risk activity due to poor judgment, such as going outside inadequately dressed, turning on only the hot water in the shower, or touching a hot stove. Patients having difficulty completing motor tasks may be at risk for falls as memory problems may lead the person to "forget" physical limitations, such as a need for assistance with ambulation or how to use a cane or crutches or use a call bell if bedridden. Some patients who are unable to judge spatial relationships may attempt to fit themselves into tight spaces, ultimately becoming trapped. The disorganized patient may also be at risk for self-harm through not eating or hydrating adequately. He may not be able to complete the steps necessary to eat a meal, forget to eat or drink altogether, or not discern food from nonfood and ingest potentially life-threatening substances. In addition, an inability to anticipate a need for toileting may result in a patient rushing to the toilet and falling or becoming incontinent and slipping.

Assessment of Risk for Self-Harm

In report. The nurse's goal is to obtain as much information about the patient's disorganized behaviors as possible in order to understand what the person is doing or may do that puts her at risk for hurting herself by accident. The nurse should specifically seek to understand current behaviors and any limitations on physical abilities. The team may brainstorm about how the patient's behavior could possibly put her at risk for self-harm in unexpected ways.

One-to-one contact. In order to assess risk of accidental injury, the nurse will conduct thorough fall risk, self-care, and physical assessments. First, with regard to *fall risk*, there are numerous fall risk scales for nurses to use, such as the Morse Fall Scale (Perell et al., 2001). These scales commonly include risk factors to look for such as: history of falls, increasing cognitive impairment, confusion, medications that increase the risk of orthostatic hypotension or may cause movement disorders, physical illnesses such as Parkinson's disease, cardiovascular or seizure disorders, use of assistive devices, and current problems such as hypotension, dehydration, and incontinence. Second, with regard to *self-care*, it is important to assess the patient's ability to meet basic needs such as toileting or expressing hunger, pain, and fatigue. The nurse will ask the patient if he would like to bathe, is hungry, is in pain, or is tired in order to observe the degree to which the patient can communicate responses verbally. Some patients will be unable to verbally communicate these essential needs. For these patients, nonverbal behaviors, such as agitation, restlessness, aggression, or combativeness may be an expression of unmet needs (e.g., pain, hunger, thirst, and/or toileting needs). Third, during the *physical assessment*, it will be important to notice any indicators of past or recent injury (bruises or burns), indicators of disease (e.g., infected wounds), or the presence of lice or scabies.

On the unit. It is essential that the nurse observe the patient's ability to walk and dress safely and to take in adequate amounts of food and fluids. Observing the patient for ability to balance, walk with steady gait, and maintain an awareness of environmental hazards will provide the nurse with additional fall risk information. Observing dressing abilities could be important as the coordinated movements required to dress oneself may create an unsafe situation. When these patients put on shoes while standing on one foot, step on the legs of the trousers, or attempt to pick up clothing from the floor, they are at risk for loss of balance and subsequent injury from a fall. Note that physical ability may fluctuate depending upon the time of day, fatigue level, and current mental status; thus, nurses should carefully note observations in the medical record and share them with other clinical team members.

● **Key Nursing Interventions to Prevent Self-Harm**

Ensure safety equipment is readily available and used. The nurse will ensure walkers and canes are available and visible, perhaps with the patient's name taped on the equipment with large letters. There are various alarm systems available to alert staff to movements of patients when risk of fall is high. Cushion alarms or motion detectors are appropriate on inpatient units when cord alarms may pose a strangulation risk.

Positioning patients at risk for falls in a chair with a safety belt allows a delay in the patient rising from the chair unnoticed. The purpose is not one of restraint, but to delay the patient long enough that the staff is able to come to the patient's assistance.

Monitor the patient closely. The nurse will have the patient at risk for falls stay in an area where the staff can monitor activity and quickly intervene if needed. Placing the patient in a room near the nurses' station, or having this person sit in a chair close to staff, allows for quick intervention when necessary.

A disorganized patient at risk for self-harm may be placed on one-to-one observation although this is an expensive and not necessarily effective mechanism to prevent falls. A staff member remaining within an arm's distance of the patient should be calm and congenial, offer gentle reminders to use a walker, and be available to help the patient regain balance if she begins to falter.

Provide assistance during bathing, dressing, and personal care. During times of personal care, the nurse will provide assistance with setting the temperature for the tub or shower. She will ensure the garments are easy to put on. Elastic or Velcro closures may be easier to use as buttons can be difficult to manage and zippers may injure a person if he pinches himself while closing it. These patients should avoid complicated clothing or items that require physical agility such as pantyhose, foundation underwear (e.g., girdles), or shoes that are difficult to put on. It may be necessary for the nurse to be present while the person is dressing. This will require a fine balance between allowing for privacy and ensuring the patient does not fall while attempting to put on underwear or socks. Some ways of maintaining privacy include having the care assistant stand to the side, avoiding extended eye contact, and maintaining light, nonpersonal conversation (e.g., about baseball, the weather, etc.).

Anticipate the patient's needs. Anticipating and preemptively meeting the patient's primary requirements will help decrease physical distress, an impending sense of urgency, and related agitation. Therefore, the nurse will anticipate basic needs, create a toileting schedule, offer snacks and fluids, encourage rest periods, and provide pain medicine when pain is suspected. The nurse should not depend upon the patient communicating these needs, as this may not be possible depending upon the level of disorganization.

Ensure adequate nutrition. The nurse will situate the patient for meal times in a setting appropriate for the patient's behaviors and with easy-to-use utensils. Staff should consider finger foods (sandwiches, cheese pieces, chicken nuggets, etc.) as these can be handled more easily by the person who has difficulty using utensils. In the vast majority of cases, safety and adequate nutrition are more important than table manners.

The nurse will open any containers of food in front of the patient, clearly describe what is on the plate, and allow some choice. The nurse may offer one-to-one help with eating as needed, but should not struggle with the patient around food or force feed at any time, as this may cause the patient to choke. Concerns about inadequate nutrition or hydration should be brought to the attention of physician.

● Subgoal: Prevent or Reduce Confrontations Between Patient and Others

In most cases, aggression for a disorganized patient is more a matter of impulsive self-protection than planned assault. The person is at risk of behaving aggressively especially during activities of daily living such as bathing or toileting. The disorganized person who is unable to understand the circumstances of another person intimately caring for him may react as if being assaulted or otherwise feel the need to protect his modesty, sometimes violently. In contrast, a patient may think an assistant is her spouse or intimate partner and attempt to reciprocate perceived affection by responding sexually. Patients may believe that they have had clothes, money, or other belongings stolen by their caregivers, laundry staff, housekeepers, and so on; this could result in aggression as well. For some patients with cognitive impairment, situations that cause embarrassment, frustration, loss of control, or loss of "face" may also stimulate an aggressive act. Finally, because a disorganized patient may demonstrate behaviors that are frightening or offensive to other people, we note that these patients are at risk for aggressive responses from others.

Assessment of Risk for Confrontations
In report. Upon hearing that a disorganized patient has acted aggressively toward others, it is important to understand the circumstances of the aggression. Finding out whom he was aggressive toward, how he exhibited aggression, and in what context will be important for identifying possible reasons why the person was aggressive. Was the aggression in the context of personal care? Did the patient believe personal property had been stolen? Did it occur at

a moment when the patient may have been experiencing intense emotions? The history of aggressive behavior is one of the most important indicators of future aggressive behavior. Identifying the person's "triggers" will allow the staff to anticipate problems ahead of time and work to diminish them. It is also important to understand and be aware of any behaviors that the patient may have that could trigger other patients to be aggressive.

One-to-one contact. It is unlikely that a disorganized person will be able to discuss aggressive behaviors or urges. Her memory of events may be unreliable. However, when interacting with the patient individually, it is wise to stay alert for indicators of increasing agitation, however minor they may seem (e.g., hand wringing, finger or toe tapping, and body tension). If the individual shows increasing agitation, the nurse should provide additional personal space and suspend the interaction if agitation continues to increase. Suspension of an interaction allows time for the agitation to dissipate and a later interaction may be more successful.

On the unit. First, the nurse should be aware of when other staff members are providing personal care to this patient, as that is a time when risk for harm to staff may be greater. When providing personal care, the nurse or staff will be on the lookout for subtle signs of mounting agitation. Second, the nurse will listen for the patient voicing concerns that personal property has been stolen. Third, the nurse will be vigilant for any situations that may heighten emotions for this patient, including shame or embarrassment. Finally, in order to prevent aggression from others, the nurse should be aware of the location and behaviors of the disorganized patient throughout the day and night and should consistently monitor patient interactions for indicators of increased agitation or socially objectionable or intrusive behavior. The disorganized patient may intrude on others by going into other patients' rooms, violating the personal space of others, or touching others inappropriately.

● Key Nursing Interventions to Prevent Aggression

Provide personal care with care. When providing personal care, how the nurse positions herself in relation to the patient is very important. When the nurse must maintain a close proximity to the patient in order to provide physical care, she must remain aware of her own personal safety. For example, a caregiver should avoid reaching across a patient as this may lead to having her breast grabbed or bitten. It is safer to assist a person with putting on shoes from the side as this may prevent a facial injury from a kick. In general, it is better for staff providing care to position themselves alongside the patient instead of in front of the person. This not only allows the staff to move away as needed but also alleviates the patient's sense of entrapment, thus decreasing the probability of assault.

Respond sensitively to a patient who claims something has been stolen. If a patient reports something has been stolen, it is important that the nurse takes the complaint seriously. The nurse will accompany the patient to the place he believes the item to have been and assess the situation and the patient's reaction. If the nurse has evidence that the item is not missing (perhaps the patient does not recognize the new clothes he's been given, or has no recollection of his items having been put in the safe), the nurse should address the affect and distress. He could say something like "I can see how upsetting this is. Is there something we can do to help you while we work this out?" He can refocus the patient as much as possible, perhaps by saying, "Can you come with me, and we will look around?" The nurse can apologize as needed: "I am sorry you do not have what you need." The nurse should not argue with the patient about the reality of the situation.

Manage heightened emotion with distraction. The staff must provide swift interventions when (1) a disorganized patient shows signs of agitation, embarrassment, or shame or (2) a disorganized patient violates social norms or behaves in a way that may provoke others. This will reduce the risk of a violent response from the disorganized patient or from other patients. In these cases, the best technique may be distraction. Distracting a patient from a potentially explosive situation can be accomplished quietly and allow for "saving face." The nurse can call the person by name, walk up to her, and ask her to come look at something, to walk with the nurse to the front desk, or to help with a task such as watering the plants or folding washcloths.

Administer medications in a way that avoids conflict. The nurse may take care to deliver medications early to patients with aggressive histories, allowing adequate time to administer medications to this patient. The nurse giving medications to this patient will want to engage the person in the process and avoid rushing the person or otherwise increasing anxiety or frustration. The process should remain congenial; the nurse should avoid struggles. The nurse can work with the patient to allow choice wherever possible. For example, a patient who objects to taking too many medications may agree to take two or three if he can leave the "rest for later." Of course, the nurse should ensure the medications that are given are of the highest priority. For example, antipsychotics or those critical to a specific medical condition may take priority over vitamins.

STABILIZATION

● **Subgoal: Decrease Disorganized Behavior and Associated Anxiety**

Anxiety and disorganized behavior may aggravate one another in a circular way, with anxiety increasing disorganized behaviors and disorganized behaviors resulting in increased anxiety (Beaudreau, 2008; Bierman, 2005; Ferreri et al., 2011; Peters, et al., 2008). Thus, interventions targeted at reducing anxiety may help decrease disorganized behavior.

Assessment of Disorganized Behavior and Anxiety
In report. Each shift will have the opportunity to gather data about the patient's ongoing level of organization over an 8-hour period, under different circumstances. The nurse will obtain information regarding the patient's ability to perform activities of daily living, communication and social behaviors, and any repetitive activities. The nurse will also want to know about observed anxiety and agitation. He will want to know about triggers for increased disorganization and anxiety, as well as a patient's previous responses to interventions intended to decrease disorganization and/or anxiety.

One-to-one contact. This contact is a good time to observe the patient's communication and social behaviors, agitation, and anxiety. The nurse can observe: How does the person respond in the conversation? What is the level of concentration and understanding? Is he able to respond to questions appropriately? Do her words make sense to him? Does he respond differently at different times of day or in different circumstances? Does she know where she is and who she is? Is there any evidence of delusions or hallucinations? Does she seem anxious or agitated?

The disorganized person may not be able to tolerate a sitting interview and the nurse should remain flexible in approach. Thus, the context of the contact may take place during an intervention such as bathing or feeding the patient, walking alongside the person while he paces, or giving medication. This allows the nurse to assess the patient's ability to conduct activities of daily living and whether the patient tends to engage in seemingly purposeless or repetitive behavior. If the person paces or moves around, it is important for the nurse to walk alongside to see if it is possible to determine the goal of the activity. How much logic does the person demonstrate as he undergoes an activity such as taking medication or dressing? Does the person spontaneously take a drink after taking the medication or is a reminder necessary?

On the unit. As described previously, the nurse will attend to the patient's ability to conduct activities of daily living and response to interventions. The nurse will also watch for seemingly purposeless or repetitive behavior on the unit. However, unless it becomes problematic, this type of behavior would not warrant intervention by the nurse. With regard to anxiety and agitation, the nurse can observe: Does the patient's level of anxiety increase or decrease at any particular time of day or in any repetitive situations? Is there a pattern to the anxiety? How often does it result in agitation or aggression?

● Key Nursing Interventions to Decrease Disorganized Behavior and associated Anxiety

Avoid overstimulation or understimulation. Overstimulation can contribute to agitation and disorganization. Thus, limiting peripheral noise and activity may prove useful. The nurse may want to turn down radios and televisions and move the patient to a quiet environment when possible. In addition, lack of sensory stimulation can also increase agitation or disorganized behavior for some people. Interventions that target the senses may increase organization. These include weighted baby dolls for the person to cuddle and hold, wrapping a person in a heated or weighted blanket, providing comfort foods such as ice cream or tea, providing soothing music, or providing familiar smells such as pies baking

(Cohen-Mansfield, 2001; Ikebuchi, 2007; Smith, 2005). Finally, many patients respond to interpersonal interaction. Making eye contact can help this patient to reorganize, even if for a short period.

Orient the person frequently. Some of the behaviors seen in the disorganized patient may be directly related to memory impairment that causes every situation to seem unfamiliar to the patient. This leads to increased anxiety and fear. Therefore, the disorganized person may require frequent orientation to time, place, and person. For example, at mealtime, the disorganized patient may think he is at a restaurant and attempt to pay the bill and leave, thus "eloping" from the inpatient unit. Quiet, gentle, matter-of-fact orientation to the environment may provide the cues necessary for the person to interact appropriately. For example, the nurse may say, "You are in the hospital dining room." The disorganized patient will also require orientation to what is happening next. This may help the patient to avoid the embarrassment of being confused. For example, at the appropriate time, the nurse may say, "It's time for dinner. Come with me."

Anticipate potentially agitating periods of time. These may include personal care times or visiting hours. The nurse may ensure the patient receives prescribed medication prior to these times to help manage anxiety. At these times, the nurse may also offer additional reassurance, provide additional distraction, or otherwise focus the person away from the agitating situation.

Encourage continuity of routines. Consistent routines, 24 hours per day and 7 days per week, will allow for a more predictable environment and minimize potential for anxiety and agitation. Discussing the routines with the patient may be helpful, but the words chosen should be easy to understand and the nurse must expect the patient's recall to be compromised to some degree. The nurse may need to frequently remind the patient of the routine.

Keep interactions and activities simple. The nurse should ask only one question at a time, maintain eye contact, speak slowly, and allow the patient adequate time to process the conversation. The nurse should also keep expectations simple, allowing small successes to provide the patient with a sense of mastery and control. He will not expect the disorganized patient to remember instructions or events that may have happened on another day.

In order to help this patient to be successful, the nurse can break down tasks that require sequential steps into simple steps and actively coach the patient at each step. This is in contrast to making requests using more complex language, such as "come with me to the dining room where you can eat dinner with other patients."

The nurse should also provide meaningful activities that do not require long periods of sustained attention or high levels of concentration. This will help to minimize frustration or agitation and give the patient a sense of accomplishment. For example, in an art group, it might be easier for this patient to color a lined picture rather than draw a picture from memory on a blank page. During a cooking group, it will be easier if one step of the recipe is assigned at a time (Smith, 2005).

Do not belittle the person. A person, especially an adult person, does not want to be treated as a child, even if she does have cognitive impairment. A nurse should never say, "What's wrong with you?" or "Here, let me do that for you." Such comments may increase the patient's agitation. Instead, the nurse may say something like, "That seems difficult for you. Would you like me to help?" or "Let's see if there is a different way to do this," when a patient has trouble accomplishing a task.

TREATMENT ENGAGEMENT

● **Subgoal: Involve the Patient in Unit-Based Activities to the Extent Possible**

Assessment of Ability to Engage in Unit Activities

A patient who is disorganized because of acute psychiatric or medical crisis (psychosis, mania, delirium) may be able to engage in the milieu activities in a progressive manner as the disorganization diminishes. Therefore, the nurse should look for changes from day to day. The nurse should start to notice improvement in ability to independently engage in activities of daily living and to communicate with others appropriately. He should start to see diminished repetitive and nonpurposeful behavior.

In contrast, the disorganized patient who is suffering from traumatic brain injury or dementia may not improve and in fact may become more disorganized. Therefore, this patient's ability to engage with members of the treatment staff and in unit activities should also be assessed on a regular basis.

● **Key Nursing Interventions to Involve the Patient in Unit-Based Activities**

Encourage participation in the milieu. The nurse will encourage a patient to participate in group activities as he is able, gauging his ability to tolerate such activity by the level of anxiety or avoidance demonstrated. The type of group activity that is appropriate may change over time. For the patient who is still quite disorganized, a sensory or exercise group may provide more benefit than an insight-oriented therapy group. If the disorganization starts to diminish, more psychotherapy-oriented groups could be more appropriate, depending on the person's cognitive abilities (Cohen-Mansfield, 2001; Ikebuchi, 2007; Smith, 2005).

Allow the patient to process any embarrassment. A patient who recompensates and begins to clear may find herself embarrassed by the disorganized behavior she has exhibited. Depending upon how much a disorganized person remembers about her behaviors, it would be beneficial for the patient to have an opportunity to discuss the experience with a nurse who is caring and nonjudgmental. Not all patients will be able to do this; however, individual needs should be taken into account. If the nurse can help the patient to feel less embarrassed about previous behavior, he may be more able to socialize and participate in activities on the unit.

PREPARATION FOR DISCHARGE

Involve the patient in the discharge process to the extent possible. Even when the patient is being transitioned to the care of others (such as family or a nursing home), it is important to include the patient in conversations about the transition. Allow the patient to participate to the extent they are able, using indicators of anxiety (e.g., fidgeting or physical agitation) to determine the time limit to the interaction. At a minimum, the nurse can clearly state what will happen: "You will be going in the ambulance to the group home." She may also reflect emotional responses back to the patient: "You look worried. Do you understand what we are saying?"

Reassure the patient. Regardless of the level of disorganization, transitions from one care environment to another can be anxiety producing. The nurse can provide reassurance that the patient will be cared for and that there will be someone to help if necessary. This will help to keep the person as calm as possible. Stating "I believe this will be a good experience for you" or "It will be alright" may be all that is necessary to provide comfort through the transition. Providing the person with a picture of the place he is going ahead of time or the written names of a person he can talk to upon arrival may also help this patient feel more secure. Sometimes sending an object from the hospital such as a magazine, a book, or even the disposable wash basin will allow the person to feel that he is taking something familiar with him to an unfamiliar place.

Provide medication education to the patient as appropriate. For the patient who is more organized at discharge, medication education and information along with ongoing community support may be appropriate. Medication information should include simple written instructions that take into account the patient's recall ability and comprehension. It may not be helpful, for example, to print out the pharmaceutical information sheet for a medication and give it directly to the patient. It would be more useful for the nurse to paraphrase the information and provide any specific instructions or precautions as bullet points.

Communicate with the next caregivers. The patient with chronic disorganization may be discharged to a nursing home or group home, or to family members with home services. The patient who has been successfully treated for psychosis, mania, or delirium may no longer be disorganized but may continue to be at risk for future episodes. Depending on the cause, the patient may be discharged to a community mental health center, a primary care provider, or an outpatient therapist. Communication between the treating team at the hospital and the outpatient providers will take place within the context of specific agency or organizational policies and procedures. It is very important, however, that helpful structures, routines, nursing actions, medications, or other interventions be shared with the aftercare services so that they can be replicated as much as possible. Inpatient staff may also want to share triggers to agitation and disorganization that have been identified. This will require clear and probably written instructions for the caregivers, family members, and any staff involved in the aftercare environment.

TABLE 3.1
Goals, Areas of Assessment, and Interventions for a
Patient With Disorganization

Goal	Assessment	Intervention
Safety		
Prevent or reduce self-harm	Assess fall risk or risk for other accidental harm	Ensure safety equipment is readily available and used
	Observe whether patient uses needed assistive devices	Monitor the patient closely
	During the physical assessment, look for indicators of past or recent injury, or disease	Provide assistance during bathing, dressing, and personal care
	Assess whether the patient has adequate food and fluid intake	Anticipate the patient's needs
	Assess the patient's ability to take care of toileting needs	Ensure adequate nutrition
Prevent or reduce confrontations between patient and others	Know past history of aggression, including context for aggression	Provide personal care with care
	Watch for increasing agitation, particularly when providing personal care	Respond sensitively to a patient who claims something has been stolen
	Watch for socially objectionable or intrusive behavior that may trigger other patients to act aggressively	Manage heightened emotions with distraction
		Administer medications in a way that avoids conflict
Stabilization		
Decrease disorganized behavior and associated anxiety	Assess patient's ability to perform activities of daily living	Avoid overstimulation or understimulation
	Observe communication and social behaviors	Orient the person frequently
	Watch for repetitive and nonpurposeful activities	Anticipate potentially agitating periods of time

(cont.)

TABLE 3.1
Goals, Areas of Assessment, and Interventions for a
Patient With Disorganization *(cont.)*

Goal	Assessment	Intervention
Stabilization		
	Observe the patient for signs of agitation or anxiety	Encourage continuity of routines
		Keep interactions and activities simple
		Do not belittle the person
Treatment Engagement		
Involve patient in unit-based activities to the extent possible	Look for day-to-day changes in level of organization	Encourage participation in the milieu
		Allow the patient to process any embarrassment

REFERENCES

Andersson, S., & Bergedalen, M. (2002). Cognitive correlates of apathy in traumatic brain injury. *Neuropsychiatry, Neuropsychology and behavioral Neurology, 15*(3), 184–191.

Beaudreau, S. O'Hara, R. (2008). Late-life anxiety and cognitive impairment: A review. *American Journal of Geriatric Psychiatry, 16(10),* 790–803.

Bierman, E. (2005). Effects of anxiety versus depression on cognition in later life. *American Journal of Geriatric Psychiatry, 13*(8), 686–693.

Chowdhury, R. F. (2003). Cognitive dysfunction in bipolar disorder. *Current Opinion in Psychiatry, 16*(1), 7–12.

Cohen-Mansfield. (2001). Nonpharmacologic interventions for inappropriate behaviors in dementia. *American Journal of Geriatric Psychiatry, 9*(4), 361–381.

Ferreri, F., Lapp, L., Peretti, C. (2011) Current research on cognitive aspects of anxiety disorders. *Current Opinion in Psychiatry 24(1),* 49–54.

Ikebuchi, E. (2007). Social skills and social and nonsocial cognitive functioning in schizophrenia. *Journal of Mental Health, 16*(5), 581–594.

Johnston, R. (2008). Evidence of semantic processing abnormalities in schizotypy using an indirect semantic priming task. *The Journal of Nervous and Mental Disease, 196*(9), 694–701.

Lippert-Gruner, K. H. (2006). Neurobehavioral deficits after severe traumatic brain injury. *Brain Injury, 20*(6), 596–574.

McCabe, R., Quayle, E., Beirne, A. D., & Duane, M. M. A. (2002). Insight global neuropsychological functioning and symptomatology in chronic schizophrenia. *Journal of Nervous and Mental Disease, 190*(8), 519–525.

Perell, K. L., Nelson, A., Goldman, R. L., Luther, S. L., Prieto-Lewis, N., & Rubenstein, L. Z. (2001). Fall risk assessment measures: An analytic review. *Journal of Gerontology: Biological Science, 56*(12), 761–766.

Peters, K., Rockwood, K., Black, S., Hogan, D., Gauthier, S., Loy-English, I., . . . Feldman, H. (2008). Neuropsychiatric symptom clusters and functional disability in cognitively impaired-not-demented individuals. *American Journal of Geriatric Psychiatry,16*(2), 136–144.

Smith, M. (2005). Behaviors associated with dementia. *American Journal of Nursing, 105*(7), 40–52.

The Patient with Manic Behavior

4

Joanne M. Matthew and Judy L. Sheehan

BACKGROUND AND DESCRIPTION

Behavior

A patient with manic behavior usually demonstrates rapid or continual movement or speech. There is often a quality of urgency in his behavior, and observers may perceive this patient as being in a state of extended physical motion, going quickly from one location to another and pacing, running, dancing, or skipping. He may seem restless, easily excited or aroused, speak in a loud voice with pressured speech, or demonstrate more subtle expressions of activity, such as tapping fingers, darting eyes, or tapping toes. This person might be easily irritated and become quickly argumentative. His pressured speech may seem frantic or jumbled and thus difficult to understand as he tries to keep up with his racing thoughts (Halter & Varcarolis, 2010). Manic behaviors are sometimes referred to as "agitation;" however, not all manic patients are agitated. Some may be jovial, flirtatious, reactive, irritated, or aroused. These behaviors can cause the patient to get into conflicts, perhaps even physical fights, with other patients, family, or visitors. Even if he is not getting into conflicts, a manic patient can "stir up" a milieu through his continual movement or other behaviors, causing other patients to become over stimulated, agitated, and distressed.

Cognition

A patient with manic behaviors may or may not have insight into the degree to which her behavior is different from others' behavior, or what is considered to be "normal" behavior. She may not understand that others do not share her sense of urgency and might instead perceive others as being "slow" or acting in an obstructionist manner. Time may be distorted for a person with manic behavior, and she may believe that the nursing staff is deliberately delaying to meet her needs, particularly for medication or meals. As a result, she may ask repeatedly, "Is it time yet?" and may react negatively to limit setting by nursing staff or other patients. Because of this distorted sense of time, this person may ask for medication, be impatient for the medication to take action, and soon declare loudly that medication doesn't work, and she wants another medication right away.

Patients with mania may have racing thoughts and flight of ideas that continuously flow at an accelerated speed. This patient may become frustrated as he speaks faster and faster, jumping from idea to idea in a pattern of disorganized speech, and perhaps becoming incoherent. The staff may have difficulty understanding him; this can frustrate him further as staff are unable to understand his needs. Staff may perceive this increased frustration as confrontational; this can lead a violent outburst on the part of the patient.

Affect

The sense of urgency experienced by this patient may cause her to feel misunderstood, ignored, extremely frustrated, and at times angry. The level of irritation may rise and fall depending upon circumstances and whether she feels thwarted in her attempts to have needs met. This level of manic activity can be exhausting for a patient, and thus she may become more irritable as she becomes fatigued (even as the level of activity interferes with sleep.)

The mood may also be labile, moving from one emotion to another rapidly with no apparent precipitant. That is, the patient may change quickly from crying to laughing, and then to being extremely irritable, and then perhaps back to laughing. At times, the person may seem euphoric, extremely enthusiastic, and giddy. He may express a sense of extreme importance and even grandiosity (Halter & Varcarolis, 2010).

Context

Obviously, manic behaviors can be seen in manic or mixed phases of bipolar disorder. However, some of the behaviors associated with a manic episode may be found in many other conditions. For example, hyperarousal and hypervigilance are symptoms sometimes seen in posttraumatic stress disorder. Psychomotor agitation can be seen in dementia and in traumatic brain injury. High activity levels may also indicate generalized anxiety disorder. Agitation can sometimes be a symptom of stimulant ingestion. An intoxicated person may demonstrate activated or manic behavior, as might a person in active withdrawal from alcohol or opiates. In these examples, arousal, activation, and mania can also be viewed on a continuum, with a person moving from an initial state of arousal to becoming more activated and then exhibiting the higher state of activation seen in manic behaviors.

A subset of patients who appear activated may in fact be experiencing akathisia. This is a distressing side effect of medications that has been defined as motor restlessness. Akathisia can sometimes be mistaken for agitated psychosis (Sharma, Madaan, & Petty, 2005).

POTENTIAL BARRIERS TO BEING THERAPEUTIC

Some of the unique issues associated with this patient apply mostly to the bipolar patient experiencing a manic episode. Specifically, the most challenging behaviors for nurses may come from the patient who is very intrusive, is grandiose, and demands staff's time. Interacting with the patient can be exhausting and responding in a consistent and therapeutic way difficult. The nurse may find the inability to satisfy this patient frustrating and may sound exasperated by the interactions on the unit and with the patient himself. This patient can be hyperobservant and will respond bluntly to any perceived ignorance, vacillation, or dishonesty on the part of the nurse. This can be a particular challenge when the nurse is trying to set limits with the patient. Further, for some nurses, witnessing or being subjected to hypersexual comments and behavior may be particularly difficult due to a history of trauma, her own cultural background or religious affiliation, or for other reasons.

OVERVIEW OF NURSING CARE GOALS

1. Safety
   - Prevent or reduce risk of accidental harm to self
   - Reduce risk of harm from others
   - Reduce risky sexual behaviors
2. Stabilization
   - Stabilize daily biorhythms and routines
   - Help patients cope with repercussions of manic behaviors
3. Engagement
   - Assist patients with engaging in treatment on the unit

SAFETY

● Subgoal: Prevent or Reduce Risk of Accidental Harm to Self

Assessment of Risk for Accidental Harm to Self

Accidental self-harm typically occurs when the patient rushes from one place to another. It can also occur when a patient is urgently trying to perform an action or task but is not using her best judgment as to how to accomplish it. In addition, it can occur when a patient does not remember or consider her physical limitations.

In report. The nurse will listen for whether the patient has shown any risky behavior such as running, standing on furniture, or not using walkers or other assistive devices.

One-to-one contact. The nurse will observe the patient's speech and motor activity for rapidity of movement. The patient may change physical positions or conversation topics rapidly. She may talk nonstop and have many ideas and thoughts to share. The nurse will want to listen for any urgent requests or needs to begin certain projects immediately as this may indicate that the patient will act without caution. This patient may be at risk for an accident due to rapid movement or poor judgment.

On the unit. It is through observation that the nurse will most likely observe the patient doing something potentially risky such as running, moving furniture, stepping on furniture to reach an object, taking apart electronic equipment, or ambulating without his assistive device. In general, the patient with manic behaviors is not likely to be someone who goes unnoticed by staff. If the patient is not active and visible in the milieu, the nurse will want to determine where he is and what he is doing to make sure he is not engaged in potentially physical risky behavior.

● **Key Nursing Interventions to Prevent Risk of Accidental Harm**

Closely supervise the patient while engaging her in safe activities. Close supervision is required to provide for general patient safety. That being said, the patient with manic behaviors, much like the paranoid patient, is going to be sensitive and reactive to close scrutiny. The close supervision of staff may be perceived as overly controlling. The challenge, therefore, is to supervise the patient closely while allowing her to engage in activities that are acceptable and that will occupy her attention and energy in a safe manner. For example, engaging the patient in craft activities outside of established group times may be useful. Staff should keep in mind that this patient may start many projects but not finish them. This patient may leave the activity midway through and then move onto the next interesting thing. The nurse will then need to ensure that the supplies are safe to be left out on the unit.

Manage the environment. This intervention involves removing or restricting access to objects or areas that are potentially dangerous to a particular patient. For example, if the patient is taking apart the electronic equipment in the sensory room, then this patient should be restricted from this area, or if the patient is taking apart the wet floor signs left by housekeeping because she needs to make a "tool" to get something out of their window, then the nurse will need to communicate the risk to other departments to make a plan. Sometimes, the plan may involve removing some of the furniture from the patient's room if the patient is standing on it or always following the patient with her assistive device if she is leaving it behind.

Provide firm limits and a consistent approach. Staff must be consistent and firm in the management of this patient and his environment. This requires effective communication to ensure that all staff members are clear about which activities are allowed and which are not. It is important to be flexible within the limits of the unit policy, so that when the nurse tells the patient what he cannot do, the nurse has an alternative activity to offer. All staff across shifts should be able to offer the same choice to the patient.

● Subgoal: Reduce Risk of Harm From Others

Assessment of Risk for Harm From Others

The risk that the patient with manic behaviors will be harmed by others is related to the level of "intrusiveness" and the particular vulnerabilities of other patients on the unit. The patient with a poor sense of personal boundaries may eventually intrude on another patient who is very irritable or aggressive, or who has poor impulse control. Consequently, the patient with manic behaviors can become the target of the other patient's anger or frustration. On a large inpatient unit, there may be a higher probability that there will be another patient with sufficient behavioral dysregulation to respond to the intrusiveness with aggression (McColm, Brown, & Anderson, 2006).

In report. The nurse will listen for staff statements that the patient has "intruded" or inserted himself into the care or visits of other patients. The nurse will also want to listen to any comments regarding telephone use, as this can be problematic for the individual with manic behaviors. For example, he may be interrupting others' calls due to the urgency he feels regarding his own need to use the telephone. Staff may mention the complaints of other patients regarding the manic patient's intrusions.

One-to-one contact. During an interaction with the manic patient, the nurse may observe that he is discussing the care or needs of other patients. He may describe how much he is helping others on the unit. The content and tone of these conversations will allow the nurse to assess the patient's focus and the level of risk present. In addition, the nurse may hear about the patient's problematic behavior during one-to-one contact or conversation with another patient and should take any information into account in order to maintain a safe environment.

On the unit. The nurse will gain the most information by observing the patient's interactions in the milieu, particularly during groups, meals, or visiting times. Some patients with manic behaviors will be seen interacting with other patients and their families. This may be due to the exclusion of her visitors or be unwelcomed attention to the other families and patients. At other times, the patient may be seen trying to assist staff and care for other patients or trying to direct the activity or care of others. Again, the nurse will want to observe who the patient is focused on and try to judge the tolerance the other patient has for the interaction.

● Key Nursing Interventions to Prevent Risk of Harm From Others

Closely supervise the patient. Close supervision may be formal or informal depending on one's organization. The nurse's assessment of the patient's level of risk and the communication of that risk to the physician will help determine what observation level is required to provide safe and adequate surveillance of this patient. In general, close supervision of the patient can be managed through whatever hospital procedures dictate observation levels. For the intrusive patient, the objective of close observation is to have staff respond quickly to refocus the patient in times when her intrusiveness is clearly bothering another patient and keep her from other patients who may harm her.

In order to monitor the intrusiveness of this patient, the nurse may want him to be in a room closer to the nurse's station. The nurse will want to communicate to other care providers a plan to keep the patient occupied and visible in the milieu. Nurses must be especially vigilant during certain times when intrusive behavior tends to increase, such as visiting hours or meal times. It can help to have the patient eat closer to the nurse's station. This will allow a nurse to step in quickly if needed.

Manage the environment. The nurse will need to decide whether an intrusive individual can participate in a particular activity or group. Often the patient who is pressured and intrusive will have difficulty in a group discussion as she tends to dominate the discussion. This potentially upsets and angers other group members. Having an alternative activity for this patient or having a staff member sit next to her in a group can be helpful.

Provide firm limits and a consistent approach. It is the nurse's responsibility to lead the team's approach to the patient and maintain consistency in the guidelines for behavior. Firm limits are needed to help protect the patient and provide containment of his behaviors. This does not mean that the patient cannot be a part of establishing some of these rules and expectations. Some flexibility will help engage the patient in the process. The challenge is to balance the patient's needs with the urgent demands that he makes (Hummelvoll & Severinsson, 2002; McColm, 2006).

The nurse should make a clear and understandable statement about the difference between appropriate and inappropriate behavior. Telling the patient clearly what she cannot do and then offering an alternative is important. For example, the nurse may say, "You cannot go into Mary's room; however, if you wish, you may …" Equally important is that all staff caring for that patient provide her with the same clear message about acceptable and safe social behavior.

It is important to consider the level of the patient's agitation when the nurse is explaining a limit. Denial of patient requests or enforcement of rules has been cited as a trigger for patient aggression (Foster, Bowers, & Nijman, 2007). Therefore, the nurse must be respectful but clear and calm when setting a limit. The nurse may want to approach the patient with other staff or be mindful of her surroundings when approaching this patient. This is also why consistency is important; a patient may become more frustrated if he receives different messages from different staff members.

Telephone use often requires limit setting as this patient may monopolize the phone or cause altercations by demanding to use it when other patients are on it. The types of limits set will depend upon unit policy. Some limits may require a physician's order; others may only need a request by a family member who is being called multiple times a day.

● Subgoal: Reduce Risky Sexual Behaviors

Assessment of Risk for Hypersexual Behavior
People with mental illness can be considered a vulnerable population and as such are susceptible to coercion. It is the nurse's responsibility to protect these patients from exploitation and the predatory behaviors of others. An individual who is demonstrating some of the behaviors associated with mania can be pursuing sexual contact with others indiscriminately. As such, it is the nurse's responsibility to protect other patients from this person's actions, as well as to protect the hypersexual individual from her own actions during a hospital stay.

Even though the inpatient unit is not a place where sexual activity is allowed, not all patients who engage in sexual behavior on an inpatient unit demonstrate hypersexual behavior. For example, some patients develop affinities for one another because of shared experiences or history. Staff may find these patients in rooms together or sitting closely in conversation. These quick connections that patients seem to make are not necessarily associated with manic behavior and may not be properly characterized as hypersexual. In this chapter, we focus only on the patient who is described as hypersexual. This patient has a higher level of libido than is normally seen, is more focused on all sexual behaviors than most patients, and exhibits impulsivity and poor judgment.

In report. The nurse may hear that the patient is making sexual comments, sitting close to other patients, or acting in a flirtatious manner. There may be reports of "intimate" or "accidental" touching of other patients or staff. There may be reports of sexual advances or suggestive comments made to the staff.

One-to-one contact. This patient may act seductively or flirtatiously with the nurse during one-to-one contact. The nurse will want to note whether the patient can be directed to discuss other topics. More overt sexual comments or conversation content that is sexualized may indicate a risk for hypersexual behavior. The nurse will need to assess the patient's ability to refocus when the conversation is directed toward other topics. If she cannot refocus or does not appreciate the inappropriateness of his comments, this may indicate that the patient is more at risk to act on her impulses. Alternatively, the patient's ability to refrain for brief periods from discussing sexual topics does not mean that she is not at any risk for hypersexual behavior.

In addition to listening to what the patient says, the nurse will be observing the patient's attire and body language as these may indicate a level of risk. For example, a patient who is at increased risk for acting on her sexual impulses may not dress appropriately or may have her genitals or breasts uncovered. Other patients may have an intense stare that appears sexualized.

On the unit. Direct observation of flirting, touching others, disrobing, or masturbating are signals of a patient at risk. The more subtle signs of attachment to another patient, such as sitting very closely together out on unit, may or may not be indicators of hypersexual behavior. The nurse will want to observe these patients and potentially investigate further.

● **Key Nursing Interventions to Reduce Risky Sexual Behavior**

Closely supervise the patient. Although this patient may need to be observed carefully, the nurse must consider the risks and benefits of having a hypersexual patient on a one-to-one type of observation. This can be difficult for the patient and staff. The patient may misinterpret the closeness and constant observation from a staff member as sexual interest. In addition, the patient may behave seductively toward the staff member. In these situations, it is important to consider what would be the appropriate gender of the staff who are watching the patient. Nursing staff assigned to this duty must be prepared to respond to flirtation or propositions from the patient. Staff must be kind, but firm when redirecting sexual comments. A patient may not remember everything that he has done when in this state, but often he will remember how staff responded and treated him.

The nurse may choose to assign this patient to a room close to the nurse's station or in a room that is not near the patient who is the object of interest. In addition, the nurse will need to assure that this patient does not spend time in rooms alone with other patients unsupervised. For example, if the unit has group rooms, sensory rooms, or lounge areas that are not easily visible to staff, this patient should not be allowed to spend time unsupervised in these areas.

Provide firm limits and a consistent approach. The nurse may need to provide frequent verbal suggestions or directives for attire and behavior. This is not an easy intervention as the patient may regard these suggestions as insulting or prejudicial. The nurse can try to say, "That is a very nice outfit for another occasion, but we want you to wear something more suitable for the hospital." However, some patients will need a more direct approach. For example, then nurse may need to say, "We expect all the patients to wear more conservative clothing."

STABILIZATION

● Subgoal: Stabilize Daily Biorhythms and Routines

Assessment of Disruption to Biorhythms and Routines
Daily routines involve specified times for eating, taking medications, being active, and sleeping or rest. For the patient with manic behaviors, establishment of routines may be particularly important (Frank et al., 2005) as his energy, attention, and state of arousal are not stable.

In report. The nurse will want to listen for any reports of the patient not eating regularly, not taking her medications, or staying up all night prior to admission. During shift report, the nurse will want to assess the same domains

- Is the patient eating during meal times? Is she taking fluids?
- Has the patient been taking her medications routinely? Is she taking only some doses and not others?
- How many hours does she sleep? When does she sleep the most? Does she sleep during the day or late afternoon but not at night? Did she sleep only an hour or less?
- Does the patient become more active or boisterous at certain times or after certain activities? Or is the patient calmer after going on walks or listening to music? How much time does the patient spend on an activity?

One-to-one contact. The nurse will want to listen for the patient's perception of the unit routines and her perception of what she needs regarding rest, food, and medications. The nurse will enquire about what and how much the patient is eating or drinking; he will ask the patient about sleeping, including how many hours and when. Also, the nurse will want to ask the patient what he did before trying to sleep. Did he listen to music? If so, what kind of music? Did he take any medications? What did he take? The nurse may ask the patient how he spent his time, that is, in groups or doing things independent of groups.

On the unit. Through observation, the nurse will also assess food and fluid intake (when, what, and how much), acceptance of medication, and sleep (when and how much). Questions to consider include: Is he having meals at the scheduled times or is he requesting food late during the night? Is she taking medication at prescribed times? Is the patient sleeping during the day, but not at night? Is the patient not sleeping at all? If the patient slept, was it after medication was administered or after a specific activity?

● Key Nursing Interventions to Stabilize Daily Biorhythms and Routines

Decrease or balance stimulation. Initially, the nurse may think that reducing stimulation is an appropriate intervention for this patient. It is possible that higher levels of noise or activity will be more destabilizing for this patient, causing him to become more hyperactive, intrusive, or agitated. However, it is not therapeutic to eliminate all stimulation. The ideal intervention is to find a balance of activity that the staff and the patient can manage. For example, loud music that has a fast beat may be too overwhelming, or certain activities can be too stimulating when engaged in all at one time (e.g., the combination of television, music, and visitors). The challenge is to find the level that keeps the patient occupied and yet still allows the patient to have some focus or self-control. The scheduling of groups and activities is important as well. In order to encourage sleep, the nurse will try to decrease the stimulation from music, television, or groups as the evening approaches.

Establish and reinforce a daily routine. Regularly scheduled times for meals, activity, sleep, and medication administration are built into the inpatient unit schedule. It is better for patients with manic behaviors to stay as close as possible to this schedule; the nurse can also remind all staff to help patient adhere to this schedule.

Although the patient with manic behaviors may benefit most from a routine with very little deviation, he may also have the most difficulty adhering to the structure and rules of the inpatient unit. When questioned, staff should present the routine schedule as beneficial to the patient. Rather than saying, "This is just how we do it," staff may say, "We are doing this in this way because we know that it will help you recover some stability."

In some instances, there may be a way to negotiate with the patient in order to get her to agree to a routine. The nurse will have to assess which requests can be reasonably accommodated. For example, a patient may want to listen to music because she finds it enjoyable. However, she might insist on listening to it at the highest volume without headphones, in the middle of the milieu, in the evening. The nurse can negotiate a more reasonable time for the patient to listen to music so that it does not disrupt the patient's sleep (by agitating her right before bed) or disrupt the experience of the other patients.

Administer medication, encourage adherence, and provide medication education. Medications for mood stabilization are essential for patients diagnosed with bipolar disorder (M. Jones & A. Jones, 2008; McColm, Brown, & Anderson, 2006; Proudfoot et al., 2009). Medication adherence has been identified as a necessary "self-management" practice for individuals with bipolar disorder (Goosens, Knoppert-van der Klein, & van Achterberg, 2008; Pollack,

1996), and medication nonadherence is one of the top difficulties for bipolar patients in the outpatient setting (Goosens, Beentjes, de Leeuw, Knoppert-van der Klein, & van Achterberg, 2008). Consequently, encouraging adherence to medication regime, providing education about medications, and helping patients to identify the benefits of medication adherence are important interventions for this patient.

Patients with manic behaviors may not want to take medications. Some may complain of side effects or the feeling of being "slowed" or sedated after taking medications. In order to discuss medication adherence, developing an alliance with the patient is important, as is providing a consistent message to the patient. The nurse should keep in mind that the patient has probably already negotiated medication type and dose with her treatment provider. If the patient starts to renegotiate medication doses or types with the nurse, it will be important for the nurse to reinforce what the patient discussed with the physician. In addition, providing education and reminding the patient that she has a choice regarding treatment may be helpful. In talking with the patient, the nurse will want to listen for indications that the patient understands the role medications may have in her recovery. The nurse can ask the patient to elaborate on this idea (i.e., that medications may be useful) in order to make the reasons that medication may be helpful and more salient in the patient's mind.

● Subgoal: Help Patients Cope With Repercussions of Manic Behaviors

This goal can be addressed as the patient becomes less intrusive, less hypersexual, or less hyperactive. The patient will likely be sleeping better and demonstrating fewer risky behaviors. She may begin to express regret about her actions. Some expert nurses conceptualize the manic state as a kind of suffering despite the euphoria some patients experience during a manic episode. As a manic state subsides, patients often feel sad about the loss of goals and relationships, as well as lonely, exposed, vulnerable, ashamed, or worthless due to the actions taken during an manic episode (Hummelvoll & Severinsson, 2002). For some individuals, there will be legal consequences, severe financial losses, and destroyed relationships in the aftermath of a manic episode. For another, the plans made for education or employment are no longer possible. Some patients lose housing due to manic behaviors. The guilt or shame the patient feels in the aftermath of the manic episode makes it more difficult to face family and associates. In addition, there may be some relationships that may not be mended.

Assessment of Readiness to Cope With Repercussions of Manic Behaviors

In report. The nurse will listen for behavioral descriptions that demonstrate a reduction in hypersexual, intrusive, or hyperactive behaviors, including unbroken sleep during the night, a longer duration of sleep, regular eating and drinking at mealtimes, attendance in group without disruption, or an overall increased participation. Perhaps the patient has been not only taking medication but also commenting on its effectiveness. These behavioral descriptions may indicate that the patient is moving to a state where he can reflect on past behaviors.

One-to-one contact. This is probably the best way to assess the improvement in the patient's ability to focus and reflect. If the patient feels that the nurse is trustworthy and nonjudgmental, the patient may comment on any regrets, guilt, or shame about past behaviors. After discharge, patients with bipolar disorder report that social and work problems are some of the top problems they experience (Goosens, Beentjes, de Leeuw et al., 2008).

Note, however, that some patients may prefer to focus on their new stability as the manic behaviors decrease. Inability to accept that one has a chronic and recurrent psychiatric disease is one of the top problems nurses encounter when working with outpatients diagnosed with bipolar disorder (Goosens, Beentjes, de Leeuw et al., 2008). Some individuals will not want to have any discussion related to regrets or past behaviors, as it may be too painful. This person should not be pushed to look at past behaviors before he is ready.

On the unit. The nurse will look for behaviors indicating a reduction in the manic episode. For example, the nurse will note the patient's ability to wait for a response to a request, a reduction in the urgency or number of requests to staff, or the occurrence of fewer intrusions on other patients during visiting or group time. At the same time, the patient will show increased ability to focus on the task at hand when in groups or on the unit. The patient may show increased interest in understanding his own treatment.

● Key Nursing Interventions to Help Patients Cope With Repercussions of Past Behaviors

Provide emotional support. This is the time to provide unconditional support, avoid recriminations, listen, and help the patient identify any supports that she has. The nurse needs to remain open to what the patient wants to express about her experience in the hospital during this episode, or about treatment in general. It is important that the nurse respond with genuine interest and concern, as well as a calm demeanor. The nurse can help the patient identify personal strengths, support her efforts to make amends for previous behaviors, rebuild healthy relationships, and help the patient to see herself as a valuable human being.

The nurse can also introduce the patient to some of the consumer support organizations in order to reduce the isolating effects of the illness and the associated stigma. Some suggestions are the Depression and Bipolar Support Alliance (www.dbsalliance.org) and the National Association for the Mentally Ill (www.nami.org).

Provide education about the patient's illness using a chronic disease model. Discussing the patient's illness using a chronic disease model may help him to reduce feelings of self-blame and consider lifestyle changes, wellness strategies, and coping mechanisms for the future. The nurse must remember to provide any information in terms the patient can understand (Goosens, Knoppert-van der Klein, & van Achterberg, 2008). Information and education must be provided incrementally as the patient's ability to focus, listen, and absorb the information improves.

Develop a relapse prevention plan. Assisting the patient in developing a relapse prevention plan can be helpful. The elements of a comprehensive relapse prevention plan include medication education, early identification of symptoms or triggers that precede a relapse or change in mood for the bipolar patient, strategies for managing specific symptoms, and general wellness skills that promote overall health (Goosens, Beentjes, de Leeuw et al., 2008; Pollack, 1996; McColm, Brown, & Anderson, 2006). Developing a relapse prevention plan is one way to help the patient focus on building a positive future instead of focusing on shame and self-blame for past behaviors. A relapse prevention plan helps the patient to feel that she may have some control over her future. While it may not be possible to develop a complete relapse prevention plan for the patient in a short inpatient stay, it is still valuable to introduce the concept and assist the patient in beginning to build a plan.

TREATMENT ENGAGEMENT

● **Subgoal: Assist Patients With Engaging in Treatment on the Unit**

Assessment of Readiness to Engage in Treatment

Each time the nurse approaches this patient to set a limit, offer medications, or assist in adhering to the unit routine, the nurse can assess the patient's willingness to engage in treatment. Initially, engagement may be nonexistent or minimal. For example, the patient might be refusing all medications, have difficulty with unit rules, or become increasingly irritable with the limits from staff. The patient may not feel ill and does not believe that he needs treatment. This person may have experienced coercive treatment during a previous hospitalization and consequently not be inclined to engage in further treatment. Frustration with being in the hospital does present a barrier to being engaged in treatment.

Another barrier to engagement is the use of the word "manic." Patients may have experienced social problems or stigma related to a manic episode and consequently will have difficulty acknowledging that they are "manic" or have "bipolar disorder." These terms may cause the patient to feel judged or criticized by the nurse. She may feel as if the nurse is calling her "crazy." It can be difficult to face the fact that one has a chronic illness and will need to take medications over the long term (Goosens, Beentjes, de Leeuw et al., 2008.)

● **Key Nursing Interventions to Increase Engagement in Treatment**

Acknowledge the patient's frustration. Sometimes, it can be helpful for the nurse to acknowledge the patient's frustration. He can convey to the patient that although it is difficult to be hospitalized, the nurse wants only to help the patient to have a positive experience. During one-to-one contact with the patient, the nurse might have the opportunity to align himself with the patient by identifying something that can be different for the patient during this hospitalization. The nurse can provide support for the patient's viewpoint and try to educate on treatment or unit routines.

Use language that the patient is comfortable with. The nurse will want to assess how the patient describes what is happening to him. When approaching the patient, the nurse may want to use words that are as neutral as possible to start with. She might say, "I notice that you have a lot on your mind, or a lot of ideas...do you think your thoughts are racing?" or "how would you describe your mood now? Is this your usual mood?" or "In the past when you have felt like this, has it caused problems for you?" Then the nurse can listen to what words the patient uses and strive to use the same language. Does the patient say that she is experiencing an episode? Does the patient describe his mood as "high," 'too high," "not myself," or "not my usual behavior?" Some patients will say, "I have trouble with my moods."

Helping the patient move toward acceptance of illness. The nurse has only a short time with this patient during an inpatient stay. It may not be possible for a person to go from a point of refusing to acknowledge that she has a long-term chronic psychiatric problem to acceptance of that she has an illness in that brief inpatient stay. However, the nurse will be helpful in the process toward recovery by being available to provide support and education to the patient and his family, encouraging adherence to follow-up appointments and encouraging the patient and the family to seek support in the community. The patient can do all of these things, potentially without labeling herself in a certain way. In addition, the nurse can help the patient see her diagnosis as similar to other chronic diseases such as asthma, diabetes, or hypertension. Like these diseases, the patient has no control over a genetic predisposition and other risk factors for illness; however, the patient can take an active role in her treatment and work to make her own life the best possible.

PREPARATION FOR DISCHARGE

For most individuals with a chronic illness, there is a need to have some basic "self-management skills." These can include medication knowledge, symptom recognition, relapse prevention, and managing emergencies and acute episodes (Pollack, 1996). It is important to have some discussions with the patient about having a plan to manage her condition. The nurse might review common types of self-management with the patient, such as taking medications, seeking spiritual strength, attending a bipolar group, finding support, seeking treatment, and avoiding substance (Pollack, 1996). In addition, the nurse can elicit the patient's own self-management or treatment preferences and assist the patient in identifying at least one intervention or activity he feels he could try after discharge. If the patient identifies an activity such as seeking volunteer opportunities or finding a support group or new learning opportunities, then the nurse can provide the patient with resources to get more information. For the patient who is experiencing financial or social losses, the nurse can advocate that the patient get referrals to any community agencies or resources that can help.

TABLE 4.1
Goals, Areas of Assessment, and Interventions for a Patient
With Manic Behavior

Goal	Assessment	Intervention
Safety		
Prevent or reduce risk of accidental harm to self	Be aware of any risky behavior, such as running, standing on furniture, taking apart electronic equipment, or ambulating without a needed assistance device	Closely supervise the patient while engaging her in safe activities Manage the environment Provide firm limits and a consistent approach
Reduce risk of harm from others	Assess patient intrusiveness with other patients Monitor telephone use	Closely supervise the patient Manage the environment Provide firm limits and a consistent approach
Reduce risky sexual behaviors	Monitor patient's sexual comments with staff or patients Watch for sexualized behavior or manner of dress	Closely supervise the patient Provide firm limits and a consistent approach
Stabilization		
Stabilize daily biorhythms and routines	Assess nutritional and fluid intake, including amount and routines for intake Monitor acceptance of medication Assess activity and sleep patterns	Decrease or balance stimulation Establish and reinforce a daily routine Administer medication, encourage adherence, and provide medication education

(cont.)

TABLE 4.1
Goals, Areas of Assessment, and Interventions for a Patient
With Manic Behavior (*cont.*)

Goal	Assessment	Intervention
Stabilization		
Help patients cope with repercussions of manic behaviors	Assess readiness to cope with repercussions of past behaviors, including decreased hypersexual, intrusive, or hyperactive behaviors, and more adherence to routines Listen for a patient expressing guilt or shame about past behaviors	Provide emotional support Provide education about the patient's illness using a chronic disease model Develop a relapse prevention plan
Treatment Engagement		
Assist patients with engaging in treatment on the unit	Assess patient's readiness to engage in treatment, that is, his ability to take medications, follow routines, follow rules, and accept limits Determine the degree to which the patient is frustrated with being on the psychiatric unit Determine whether the patient is able to accept that he has a psychiatric illness	Acknowledge the patient's frustration Use language that the patient is comfortable with Help the patient move toward acceptance of illness

REFERENCES

Foster, C., Bowers, L., & Nijman, H. (2007). Aggressive behavior on acute psychiatric wards: Prevalence, severity and management. *Journal of Advanced Nursing, 58*(2), 140–149.

Frank, E., Kupfer, D. J., Thase, M. E., Mallinger, A. G., Swartz, H. A., Fagiolini, A. M., ... Monk, T. (2005). Two year outcomes for interpersonal and social rhythm therapy in individuals with bipolar I disorder. *Archives in General Psychiatry, 62*(9), 996–1004.

Goosens, P. J. J., Beentjes, T. A. A., de Leeuw, J. A. M., Knoppert-van der Klein, E. A. M., & van Achterberg, T. (2008). The nursing of outpatients with bipolar disorder: What nurses actually do? *Archives of Psychiatric Nursing, 22*(1), 3–11.

Goosens, P. J. J., Knoppert-van der Klein, E. A. M., & van Achterberg, T. (2008). Coping styles of outpatients with a bipolar disorder. *Archives of Psychiatric Nursing, 22*(5), 245–253.

Halter, M. J., & Varcarolis, E. M. (2010). Bipolar disorders. In E. M. Varcarolis & M. J. Halter (Eds.), *Foundations of psychiatric mental health nursing* (pp. 280–303). St. Louis, MO: Saunders Elsevier.

Hummelvoll, J. K., & Severinsson, E. (2002). Nursing staff's perceptions of persons suffering from mania in acute psychiatric care. *Journal of Advanced Nursing, 38* (94), 416–424.

Jones, M., & Jones A. (2008). Promotion of choice in the care of people with bipolar disorder: A mental health nursing perspective. *Journal of Psychiatric and Mental Health Nursing, 57,* 87–92.

McColm, R., Brown, J. & Anderson, J. (2006). Nursing interventions for the management of patients with mania. *Nursing Standard, 20,*(17), 46–49.

Pollack, L. E. (1996). Inpatient self-management of bipolar disorder. *Applied Nursing Research, 9*(2), 71–79.

Proudfoot, J. G., Parker, G. B., Benoit, M., Manicavasagar, V., Smith, M., & McCrim, A. G. (2009). What happens after diagnosis? Understanding the experiences of patients with newly-diagnosed bipolar disorder. *Health Expectations, 12,* 120–129.

Sharma, A., Madaan, V., & Petty, F. (2005). Propanolol treatment for neuroleptic-induced akathisia. *The Primary Care Companion to the Journal of Clinical Psychiatry, 7*(4), 202–203.

The Patient With Nonsuicidal Self-Injury

5

Joan S. Kovach

BACKGROUND AND DESCRIPTION

Over the years, the prevalence of self-injurious behaviors in the United States has been on the rise (Walsh, 2008), and the understanding of these behaviors has grown and changed. Although patients who self-injure are 18 times more likely to commit suicide than those who do not self-injure (Van Sell et al, 2005), nonsuicidal self-injury (NSSI) is different in many ways from suicidal behavior. Unlike suicidal behavior, NSSI is associated with the following: no intent to kill oneself and therefore less potential lethality; less intense feelings of psychological pain, hopelessness, or helplessness; and the presence of a typical pattern of events leading up to the NSSI that is specific for each patient. For instance, a patient may be getting ready to go somewhere, and when she glances in the mirror, she sees herself in a negative way. She begins to feel inferior and unlovable. This triggers the well-rehearsed, often-used behavioral response of taking her comb and scratching the inside of her forearms until they bleed. This causes the intense feelings of inferiority to somehow be relieved. The level of risk of the behavioral response may be low (using a comb) or high (cutting with a blade). Whereas there are times when lethality results from NSSI (Van Sell et al., 2005), it is understood that suicide had not been the patient's goal.

Patients often have difficulty reducing or eliminating NSSI, and there is always a possibility of relapse. Walsh (2008, p. 3) acknowledges that self-injury is often a "strangely effective coping behavior, albeit a self-destructive one." Consistently throughout the literature, self-injurious behaviors are described as the actions of a person who seeks to shift "overwhelming emotional pain to a more acceptable physical pain" (Hicks & Hinck, 2008, p. 409). A second function of self-injurious behavior may be a social one. "NSSI may be especially likely when other communication strategies have failed…" (Nock, 2009, p. 3). It is critical to understand that NSSI serves an important purpose for patients seeking relief from emotional or psychological pain.

Behavior

NSSI is defined by Walsh (2008, p. 4) as "intentional, self-effected, low-lethality bodily harm of a socially unacceptable nature." Self- injurious behaviors include acts such as rubbing, cutting, carving, punching, burning, pinching, pulling at one's skin or hair, swallowing dangerous objects or substances, and any behaviors that result in self-induced physical injury. Self-injury that is not life threatening, that does not pose a serious threat to physical health, and that requires minimal or no first aid is considered "mild." In this case, treatment of the physical wound can safely be self-administered. Self-injury that results in bodily harm, that requires immediate medical assistance, or that poses a serious threat to immediate or future health or well-being is considered "severe."

Behaviors considered "socially acceptable," such as ear piercing, are not considered NSSI. However, there is a grey area in which certain behaviors are socially acceptable in some cultures but not in others. For example, intentional scarring of the face and body may be considered NSSI in the United States, but it may be normative in certain

African tribes (http://www.everyculture.com/Sa-Th/ Sudan.html#ixzz1XhNACBlW [under: *Symbols of social stratification*]).

Cognition

Patients with NSSI may tend to interpret ambiguous life events in a very negative way. When these beliefs are associated with "unbearable emotional distress and impaired coping skills with which to alter the situation..." (Hicks & Hinck, 2007, p. 410), self-injury may result. For example, a patient may make a phone call to a friend for support and the friend does not answer. The patient interprets this to mean that her friend is avoiding her and does not like her, triggering overwhelming feelings of rejection and isolation. The patient may then go to her room, find a paper clip, and scratch her arm until it bleeds. The patient may have the desire to stop self-injurious behaviors while still performing them. Distortions in thinking are often present in those who self-injure (Beck, 2005). These distortions include the following:

All–or–nothing thinking. A person, an event, or an experience is evaluated in an extreme way: as either good or bad, or as representing perfection or failure. There is no middle ground. For instance, a patient thinks, "I'm really great at this" or "I'm a total failure at this." The possibilities of being "pretty good" or "not too bad" do not exist.

Mind reading. This refers to the condition in which a patient assumes she knows what other people are feeling and thinking, especially as it relates to herself. For instance, the patient thinks, "I know that she is thinking I'm stupid and I will never be good at this." Even if the other person were to honestly deny evaluating the patient in this way, it does not usually provide relief. The patient believes that she knows better and can read the other person's mind.

Emotional reasoning. Patients may believe that an experience of emotion must always reflect an underlying truth rather than a passing feeling. For instance, the patient feels something is wrong so it must be wrong: "I feel anxious and so there must be something to be anxious about. I'm sure it's that no one will be coming to visit me tonight." While the patient is correct about her anxious feeling, she has no data about whether or not someone will visit. The experience of anxiety dominates her reality, and she may make incorrect predictions about what is happening or what will happen based on the fact that she is anxious.

Affect

In many cases, patients who self-injure suffer from both an inability to accurately name and describe strong affect and an inability to manage it. Affect is often experienced as very intense and may include anger, sadness, hopelessness, helplessness, shame, guilt, and feelings of loss and abandonment that sweep in and take over quickly. Sometimes, there is a state of dissociation or emotional numbness. When emotions are intense and overwhelmingly painful, patients say that self-injury can provide short-term relief, although it ultimately may lead to more pain, shame, or self-hate (Hick & Hinck, 2007).

Context

Patients with self-injurious behavior on the inpatient unit can have a myriad of additional coexisting problems and single or overlapping diagnoses. Individuals with personality disorders (most consistently, borderline personality disorder), posttraumatic stress disorder, anxiety, eating disorders, dissociative disorder, major depressive disorder, obsessive–compulsive disorder, somatoform disorder, and psychotic disorders can all have NSSI.

Originally thought to occur mainly in incarcerated or mentally ill populations, self-injury has emerged in youth in middle and high schools, in adolescents and young adults in colleges, and in adults in the general population (Walsh, 2008). Young, Sweeting, and West (2006) found that one group of adolescents known as "Goths" or "Emo" appears to have a higher rate of self-injurious behaviors. Their study suggests that young people who self-injure identified themselves as Goths because they felt that their emotional distress would be understood in this subculture. This study did not find that peer pressure was a cause of self-injury. However, Walsh (2008) stresses the crucial importance of peer pressure. He states, "If a small circle of friends stop self-injuring, an individual may give it up with or without treatment." He also stresses that there is a growing number of self-injuring adolescents who are healthier psychologically and who give up the behavior more easily than those with complicating mental illnesses.

In the case of psychosis, although self-injury is self-inflicted, the intentionality is in question because it may be in response to voices—command hallucinations or self-deprecatory comments—which the patient cannot control. In the case of developmental disabilities, including autism, mental retardation, and brain injury, self-injury may include repetitive behavior, such as head banging, self-scratching, biting, picking, or hitting, that occurs at a high rate of frequency. Simeon and Favazza (2001) observe that it is "fixed, contentless, and driven" and describe it as stereotypic self-injury. Both psychotic self-injury and the stereotypic self-injury of the cognitively impaired requires a more specialized nursing intervention to protect the patients' safety than in the case of patients who do not have these problems. These patients may not be responsive to cognitive types of interventions. Instead, the nurse will have to focus on managing the environment to reduce triggers and to reduce access to means. In the case when serious self-injury (such as head banging) is already in process, protection from self-harm requires more active intervention by the nurse up to and including physical, mechanical, and/or chemical restraint.

POTENTIAL BARRIERS TO BEING THERAPEUTIC

Care of the patient with NSSI poses particular challenges for the nurse. Most nurses go into the profession to relieve suffering and to help patients in their journey to wellness. It can be baffling to meet patients who self-injure and difficult to come to any empathic understanding of why anyone would do this. Often, these patients are physically attractive, stylish, and professionally competent, and it may seem incongruous that they have serious mental health issues. Anger at these patients is not uncommon as they seem to thwart the nurse's efforts and frustrate his attempts to support them and protect them from injury. In addition, it is easy and tempting for a nurse to feel that there is an opportunity to be special, to be the one person this patient trusts, and to be able to save the patient from herself. Staff so easily find themselves split over how they see a self-injurious patient, and nurses can feel very hurt or like a failure when a patient is unable to honor a promise or plan made with a nurse. Therefore, it is imperative that the nurse working with patients with NSSI

- Accepts that these patients are suffering and the self-injury is often an attempt to relieve that suffering
- Understands that some of these patients have experienced disturbed or distorted relationships and have little experience of a trusting relationship and therefore may not have skills needed to build a trusting relationship
- Learns the merits of such nursing interventions as *emotional nonresponse* or maintaining strict *consistency*. These

are interventions that at first may feel wrong, uncaring, or unnatural

OVERVIEW OF NURSING CARE GOALS

1. Safety
- Prevent unintentional lethality from NSSI
- Reduce frequency and severity of NSSI

2. Stabilization
- Identify and decrease the distress that is an antecedent of NSSI
- Assist patient in learning and using alternative coping skills

3. Engagement
- Increase engagement in treatment and trust in treatment providers

SAFETY

● **Subgoal: Prevent Unintentional Lethality From NSSI**

Increased risk for NSSI also represents increased risk for unintentional lethality. Assessment and interventions for NSSI more generally will be discussed in the next section. Here, we focus specifically on assessment and management of specific behaviors that can possibly result in lethality.

Assessment of Risk for Unintentional Lethality

In report. In order to assess risk for unintentional lethality while on the unit, the nurse will listen for the following information:

- Does the reason for this hospitalization include a serious suicide attempt or NSSI (without intent) that could have been lethal? For example, many people do not think of aspirin or acetaminophen as being as dangerous as prescription medications when used to overdose. However, death can eventually result from internal bleeding or liver damage. Speeding and the resultant car crash are frequently portrayed in the entertainment media as a nonlethal dramatic event with a hospitalized and hopeful protagonist in the final scene. Therefore, patients may not view speeding as lethal. In fact, immediate fatalities or eventual deaths from sustained injuries are far more common than anticipated.

- What were the external events that precipitated the behavior? For instance, health problems, especially cancer of the head and neck, HIV/AIDS, multiple sclerosis, and epilepsy are known to increase suicide risk (Hawton, 2000). Potentially life-changing and irreversible events, such as catastrophic financial losses, or any losses that involve shame are more likely to precipitate suicide attempts compared with repetitive troubles (Kalafat & Lester, 2000). Have there been any such problems or events reported by the patient or family?
- What are the patient's thoughts about the possibility of dying? Is there any ambivalence about living, which, combined with impulsivity and a history of NSSI, poses an increased risk?
- What are this patient's recent and remote suicide attempts (if any)? Is there any family history of suicide? What is the status of the patient's feelings of hope or hopelessness? What is his future orientation? Does he have a history of impulsivity?

A history of medically serious self-injury without intent to kill oneself, ambivalence about living, past suicide attempts, family history of suicide, hopelessness, or impulsivity increase the risk of unintentional lethality from self-injurious behavior. NSSI is a very strong predictor of having a future successful suicide attempt (Hawton, 2009).

"Parasuicide is an established risk factor for eventual suicide" (Comtois, 2002, p. 1139).

As the patient's inpatient stay progresses, the nurse will also want to hear how the patient has managed safety and impulsivity on previous shifts. In report, staff can communicate whether a patient has made any threats to hurt himself through hanging, ingesting toxins, or cutting himself using items found on the unit.

One to one. In addition to assessing risk for self-injurious behavior, more generally, the nurse will want to assess risk specifically for nonintentional lethality. That is, the nurse will ask the patient the following:

- Has the patient been thinking differently about self-harm? For example, the patient who usually scratches herself may start to describe how she would use her bathrobe and the door to hang herself to get relief from her distress. Or, she may admit that she had asked her friend to smuggle her some medication so she can overdose.
- How does the patient report her mood and what do staff observe about her mood? Has there been any increase in sadness, despondency, frustration, anxiety, or agitation since the patient came onto the unit?
- Are there any new events in her life that might trigger serious NSSI or suicide attempts?
- Has the patient had any thoughts of suicide? What does she believe is the risk that she will harm herself now and throughout the next shift?

Other causes for concern that the nurse may notice during the one-to-one interaction include avoidance of eye contact, reports of uncontrollable urges, and avoidance of discussion of recent losses or suicidal feelings.

On the unit. The nurse will continue to assess for risk of unintentional lethality.

- What is the status of environmental safety? Are there any cords or sharps on the unit to which the patient has access?
- While in the milieu, has the patient evidenced any signs of increased agitation, as demonstrated by noncompliance with unit rules, yelling or increased volume when speaking, disregard for the wellbeing of other patients, blocking a door, or throwing items?
- Is the patient less visible than usual? Is she isolating in her room? Are others reporting secretive behaviors? What about secretive interactions with visitors? These behaviors are of particular concern if they represent a new behavior for the patient.

● Key Nursing Interventions to Decrease Risk of Unintentional Lethality

Increase level of observation. There are a few ways to do this. First, if the nurse has reason for concern about patients who are a high risk for serious self-harm, she can increase frequency of checks according to the policy at her hospital. Second, the nurse can request or insist that the patient stay in open, visible areas. Sometimes, this involves a reverse room plan so that the patient stays out of her room for long stretches of time; a patient's bedroom door can be locked to help enforce reverse room plan. Third, if appropriate, the patient can be moved to the room with roommates and/or closer to the nurses' station. This decreases opportunities for isolation.

Explore ambivalence and understand impulsivity. The nurse can use one-to-one time to explore the patient's level of impulsivity and allow the patient to express ambivalence about living and dying. If the patient is impulsive, or has a lot of self-harm thoughts or wishes for death, she is at higher risk for unintentional lethality. Therefore, if the patient wishes, the nurse can give her a safe space to express suicidal thoughts and emotional pain. Once the patient expresses the thoughts, the nurse has a chance to tell the patient that it is okay to have these thoughts and that the patient does not need to act on them even if she has them. Further, the nurse can then explore ambivalence. The nurse can give the patient an opportunity to express all their reasons for dying, as well as reasons for living. A patient may begin by saying that it would not matter to anyone if she died. The nurse may then encourage her to think about this carefully, and in particular to think about how family members, pets, or others may react to her suicide. As the patient does this, she may see some reasons for living. Another reason for living may be that dying does not help to express her feelings but instead silences them. As the nurse listens to the reasons for living and dying, she makes efforts to reinforce reasons for living by paying special attention to them ("What are your grandchildren's names? How old are they?"). It is challenging for a nurse to have this conversation and remain neutral and unalarmed, but very helpful to patients. This type of conversation shows how it can be safe to talk and think about something (suicide) without acting on it.

Ensure environmental safety on the unit. The nurse will make sure that basic rules of unit safety are observed. He will check for any risky exceptions to the normal precautions for safety. Sometimes, there may be maintenance staff on the unit with tools that are dangerous and accessible to patients. Perhaps, a patient being discharged has belongings, including sharps, packed and waiting by the door. The nurse will reinforce rules with staff and be vigilant about dangerous items on the unit. The nurse and team should try to think creatively about what types of objects a patient may use for self-injury. For example, a patient could cheek and save meds to get enough for an overdose, and therefore require mouth checks. Another patient could collect and drink the hand sanitizers provided. These materials would need to be removed from the unit until this behavior is eliminated. Every environment has potential safety challenges. The nurse will work to recognize and minimize these on the unit.

Use restraint as a last resort. Restraint is used only when the patient is in danger of serious injury, and no other interventions to stop or prevent the self-injury are working. One such scenario could be a patient with persistent head-banging. When the nurse and other staff use physical restraint, they are always clear that the intervention is about patient safety, and that the patient is informed that the restraint is to help him stay safe and uninjured. All institutions have policies on the use of restraint and seclusion, as well as training in de-escalation, to help reduce the need for restraint. By staying familiar with these policies, nurses ensure that the infrequent, but necessary, episodes of restraint and/or seclusion will be carried out safely and in accordance with the established guidelines.

● **Subgoal: Reduce Frequency and Severity of NSSI**

Assessment of NSSI
In report. During the initial report, the nurse will listen for the following information to understand the frequency and severity of NSSI:

- History of illness: What were this patient's self-injurious behaviors over the course of her illness? Prior to admission, what was the frequency and severity of her NSSI?
- Since admission, have there been episodes of NSSI or close calls? What nursing interventions occurred and what were the results? Did increased one-to-one time relieve impulse to self-injure, or did the behavior increase

when the one-to-one ended? Did the medication help? What other interventions helped?

- Have there been any episodes of increased anxiety or agitation during the previous shift? If so, what interventions were offered and what were the results? Did the patient use prn medications or music or other self-soothing interventions, or talk with staff? Did any of these help? The response to the treatment in the previous shift will help the nurse understand and evaluate the efficacy of the current care plan.

- Has the patient expressed any interest in decreasing the self-injurious behaviors? Are the behaviors ego-syntonic, that is, experienced as "normal" by the patient?

- Is the patient on the unit of her own accord? If her parents or school requires that she gets the treatment, she may not have an interest in decreasing NSSI. If so, what are the patient's goals for being on the unit? Is she studying other patients to learn about self-injury, and therefore is in danger of increasing frequency and severity of NSSI?

One-to-one contact. The nurse can directly ask the patient about NSSI and potential antecedents to NSSI. This direct inquiry sets the tone for collaboration. The nurse may ask

- Have there been recent events on the unit that might be a precipitant to NSSI? How did the patient manage these events?

- Has the patient noticed any urges to self-injure? Can he come to staff for help if she has these urges?

- What is the patient's affect: is there any increase in sadness, despondency, frustration, agitation, or anxiety?

- Has the patient recently engaged in self-injury? If so, the nurse will ask the patient to allow the nurse to see it.

- What does the patient plan to do to keep himself safe?

On the unit. The nurse will continue to assess the safety of the milieu and patient's progress in decreasing the incidence of and severity of NSSI.

- Has there been any change in the interactions with other patients?
- Has there been any contraband discovered on the unit that is potentially relevant?
- Is there any increased isolative behavior, secretive behavior, or illogical behaviors—such as changing to long sleeves on a hot day—indicating hidden marks and increased risk for NSSI?

● **Key Nursing Interventions to Decrease Severity and Frequency of NSSI**

Negotiate an agreement that the patient will inform staff if she feels at risk of self-harm. Safety contracts have been shown to be of limited value in preventing self-injury (Shea, 1999) and often cause patients feelings of shame and failure. They simply ask the patient to give up one way of coping without ensuring that another is in place. Therefore, we do not recommend using only a traditional "safety contract" in which the patient is asked not to self-injure. Instead, staff will talk with the patient and make a request that the patient go to staff when she has urges to self-injure. The patient will know that staff can then offer medication to reduce urges, increase safety orders, offer one-to-one time to help identify feelings associated with urges, and offer other distractions.

Offer prn medication. As the nurse and patient begin to understand some of the subjective experiences that are precipitants to NSSI, they may design a plan to use medication to assist in managing these experiences. Typical medications include antipsychotics, benzodiazepines, and other anxiolytics. Initially, the nurse can offer prn medications for symptoms of agitation or anxiety. However, the nurse may observe that scheduled medications work better than prn medications for the patient because the patient is not yet able to recognize her need for medication in a timely manner. The nurse can then work with the physician to change the orders to standing medications for a time.

Utilize sensory interventions. Sensory interventions have been shown to assist with management of anxiety and other overwhelming sensations (Knight et al., 2010). The nurse can orient patients to and offer activities such as holding a frozen orange, sucking on sour candies, wearing colored sunglasses, using a weighted blanket and/or rocking chair, practicing deep breathing, and using aroma therapy. These may help to decrease risk of self-harm.

Have a plan for what will happen should the patient engage in self-harm. An agreement between the patient and staff can also include predictable consequences of engaging in NSSI on the unit. Staff can make NSSI actions inconvenient so that the patient begins to feel it takes more effort to manage feelings using NSSI than using other available coping mechanisms. That is, following a NSSI, the patient may be asked to discuss with staff the precipitants, experiences, and actions involved in NSSI. Staff may use a tool to help the patient analyze problem behavior to do this (e.g., see Marsha Linehan's *Skills Training Manual for Treating Borderline Personality Disorder*). Other consequences of NSSI may be that the patient is obligated to stay in open areas or to spend time in front of the nurses' station, and is ineligible for certain privileges. Because some of these consequences can feel punitive, it is key that they are negotiated with the patient ahead of time.

Part of the agreement that the patient and staff negotiate may include the fact that staff will minimize their emotional response to NSSI incidents. This allows staff to address the severity of the injuries while at the same time not reinforcing the NSSI by associating it with desired increases in staff attention. Nursing care can take the form of *emotional nonresponse with no action*, in which NSSI and ensuing minor injuries are ignored, or *emotional nonresponse with some action*, which consists of a standard set of actions (that all staff use). These actions may include acknowledging the injury and initiating planned sequelae. Emotional nonresponse is sometimes referred to as *benign neglect*. It is in fact not neglect, but a carefully chosen response. It is effective for patients who have come to believe (consciously or not) that their main source of attention and validation comes after self-injury. When using emotional nonresponse, staff interact normally with the patient around other events such as meals, groups, setting goals at community meeting, or efforts in exercise group, but change their affect around self-injury to one of nonresponse, and their actions to an underresponse.

We provide here some sample plans for consequences of NSSI. For patients with mild NSSI, that is, injuries requiring no medical interventions, the nursing response is understated. The nurse may say, "Why don't you sit here while I get a band aid?" "How do you feel about this?" "What can you do that would be different next time?" With this type of response, the nurse can place the responsibility of the action back on the patient. Restricting the patient environment may not be necessary as a response to an episode of mild NSSI.

The plan for responding to injuries that are more severe and/or potentially life threatening is different. First, those providing nursing or medical care do so with decreased emphasis on first aid and increased emphasis on behavioral analysis. For example, while dressing a wound, the nurse will not discuss the physical injury, but will stay focused on the need for the patient to think about the pros and cons of the behavior. The patient may be expected to assist with dressing the wound in order to promote responsibility for his own actions. Second, a staff member will implement agreed-upon restrictions necessary to keep the patient safe, such as discontinuing off-unit privileges (as the patient cannot demonstrate the ability to stay with the group.)

Establish an appropriate level of supervision. Depending on recent history, the nurse will modify observation level for the patient. If the patient's responses indicate an inability to control urges or if there is report or discovery of new injuries despite the patient's agreement to report urges to self-injure, and if the injuries are potentially severe, the nurse will want to increase the level of surveillance. Utilizing the least restrictive measures possible, the nurse will help patients maintain self-control by offering activities in open areas (e.g., coloring, reading, music, journaling). However, if episodes of NSSI persist frequently, the nurse may need to ensure that the patient stays in open areas, use a reverse room plan, increase the frequency of checks, or put the patient on self-checks. The latter is a system that has the patient return to a designated spot every 15 minutes to sign in. This allows for increased observation without the secondary gain of increased staff attention, which might unintentionally reinforce the NSSI.

Employ room changes. On units with shared patient rooms, the composition of the group of roommates can affect patients' efforts to decrease NSSI and nurses' efforts to teach alternate behaviors to patients. Nurses should be conscious of alliances between patients who support the treatment and those who work against the treatment goals. Different patients may have different perspectives on the use of self-injury, and judicious room changes can be employed to interrupt a nonsupportive relationship or to foster a relationship in which patients support one anothers' goals and treatment.

Note and acknowledge any decreased frequency or severity of NSSI. If possible, the nurse will identify any decrease
in NSSI since the previous contact. This may be done in
the context of the one-to-one contact. Acknowledging
and appreciating the patient's use of appropriate coping
skills may assist the patient with motivation for change.
For example, rather than focusing on recent scratches to
the wrist, the nurse can comment that the patient has been
honoring her agreement to seek out staff for help when
she has urges to self-injure and has been going for longer
stretches without NSSI.

STABILIZATION

● Subgoal: Indentify and Decrease the Distress That Is
  an Antecedent of NSSI

Assessment of Patient's Experiences of Distress
In report. During report, the nurse will listen for episodes
of distress for the patients. In the last 24 hours, have there
been any noted episodes of NSSI? If so, what were the precipitating events? Is there any new knowledge of what
experiences cause the patient high levels of emotional
distress?

One-to-one contact. During the one-to-one contact, the
nurse will explore the patient's recent experiences of distress. She might start with a question such as, "Since we
spoke yesterday, have you had any situations that were
upsetting to you?" After identifying distressing episodes,
the nurse will ask the patient if he can identify any progress (in groups and individual work) on the recognition
of symptoms that are early signs of growing distress. The
nurse may also compare how the patient talks about distress in this contact to how the patient has talked about
distress previously. The nurse will consider whether the
patient is developing an increased capacity to name his

feelings. Finally, the nurse will inquire whether the patient has any examples of detecting experiences that often precede increasing distress (i.e., "triggers"). These questions may reveal increasing insight and point to particular situations in which patients need help in managing distress.

On the unit. The nurse will be tuned in for signs of escalating levels of distress. This could be a raised voice, arbitrary oppositional behavior or demands, persistent requests for medication or staff attention, patient conflicts, or provocative family meetings. The nurse will attend to how the patient managed this distress. Does she revert to NSSI? Or, does she use sensory interventions or other healthy coping techniques taught on the unit?

● **Key Nursing Interventions to Help Patients Identify and Reduce Distress**

Help patients identify emotions that may trigger impulses for NSSI. A patient may already have been presented with the grid of emotions (see Figure 5.1). Using this emotion chart or a similar one, the nurse asks the patient to choose words that best describe her feelings. The patient may identify with the word *glum*, rather than *depressed* or *sad*; with *agitated* or *edgy* rather than *fearful*; with *irritable* rather than *angry*; or with *mortified* rather than *shamed*. We note that the emotion of joy, while pleasant, can also be difficult for a patient because the patient may have had the repeated experience of a joyful feeling quickly followed by feelings of fear or loss.

Then, as difficult subjects are discussed and the patient experiences stressful emotions, the nurse will ask the patient if she can name these emotions. The nurse will also assess the level of distress as evidenced by nonverbal clues like changes in posture or affect, or the patient's attempt to to avoid a subject. The nurse can then help the patient recognize what is happening. By participating in

SADNESS

Abandoned	Demoralized	Desperate	Hurt
Alone	Dejected	Empty	Lonely
Awful	Depressed	Excluded	Melancholy
Agonized	Despairing	Forsaken	Miserable
Anguished	Disappointed	Fragile	Mournful
Battered	Discontented	Glum	Sad
Blue	Dismayed	Grief Stricken	
Crushed	Distraught	Hopeless	
Defeated	Discouraged	Helpless	

FEAR

Afraid	Disconnected	Helpless	Restless
Agitated	Distracted	Horrified	Scared
Alarmed	Disturbed	Hysterical	Shocked
Anguished	Dread	Insecure	Shaky
Anxious	Edgy	Nervous	Terrified
Confused	Fearful	Numb	Uneasy
Dazed	Frightened	Overwhelmed	Worried
Defensive	Frustrated	Panicked	

ANGER

Angry	Critical	Hateful	Rebellious
Aggravated	Disgusted	Hostile	Reckless
Agitated	Displeased	Irritable	Revengeful
Aggressive	Disturbed	Impatient	Scornful
Annoyed	Exasperated	Loathing	Spiteful
Belligerent	Enraged	Opposed	Unfriendly
Bitter	Envious	Outraged	Vicious
Contemptuous	Furious	Resentful	
Combative	Harsh	Revulsion	

SHAME / GUILT

Shamed	Foolish	Jealous	Ridiculous
Accountable	Humiliated	Minimized	Regretful
Awkward	Ignored	Mocked	Remorseful
Culpable	Inferior	Mortified	Scorned
Defective	Insulted	Neglected	Self-reproachful
Embarrassed	Invalidated	Responsible	

FIGURE 5.1 Red Flag Emotions. (*continued*)

JOY

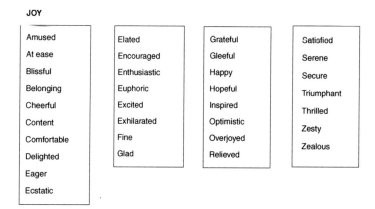

FIGURE 5.1 Red Flag Emotions. (*continued*)
Source: The Proctor House II Coping & Crisis Plan Packet,
property of McLean Hospital.

this activity, the patient begins building skills of knowing her own emotions. This is the first step toward the patient being able to identify times when she needs to proactively engage in adaptive coping skills to avoid NSSI.

Validate the patient's feelings. With respect for the patient's report of the distress, the nurse will acknowledge the feeling and the patient's right to have that feeling, and suggest they work together to manage the distress. For example, a patient who feels slighted by another patient might have a mild feeling of loneliness accompanied by a sense of distress and the urge to scratch her wrist for relief from it. If the nurse can validate the feelings of loneliness and distress, he may make the feelings more tolerable and acceptable, as well as suggest ways to cope with the feelings. Unchecked and unacknowledged, the feeling can escalate to mortification and be accompanied by thoughts of being defective. Also, a patient may believe that she should not have a certain feeling. This is a belief that only increases distress. As feelings become more overwhelming, urges to inflict self-injury for relief may intensify.

The nurse should be aware that comments like "just calm down" or "just relax" can be experienced as dismissive and invalidating. Dismissing the feeling leaves the patient voiceless and searching for a way to express and relieve the pain. The patient may also feel the need to *prove* how bad she feels.

Remind the patient that feelings cannot be avoided but can be managed. The nurse can teach the patient that it is the feelings that are not accepted or are pushed away that produce deeper distress that may be antecedent to impulsive behavior. For example, if a patient says to himself, "I can't stand feeling this way" or "I shouldn't feel this way," this creates additional distress. The nurse can listen carefully, and model acceptance of feelings by saying "It's okay if you feel this way" or "given what has happened, it makes sense that you feel this way." When he does this, the nurse will want to manage his own facial expression so that he truly looks accepting, rather than fearful or disgusted. The nurse can then go on to say, "Let's think about how to manage the feeling. You don't have to hurt yourself because you feel this way. Let's discuss other options."

Help patients identify other triggers for urges to self-injure. These may be behaviors, thoughts, bodily sensations, and actions. Sometimes patients feel that their urge to self-injure comes "out of the blue." In fact, a careful review of preceding events may result in the identification of types of situations that can be distressing and trigger urges to NSSI. The nurse may ask the patient, "What were you doing just before you cut yourself?" "What was happening?" "Where were you?" "What was happening around you?" "What was going through your head?" Examples of experiences that can be distressing include:

- Awaiting a visitor or family meeting on the unit. Upon questioning, the patient may say he was feeling afraid that they would not come and he would feel rejected.
- Receiving a phone call from her family. This could cause the patient to feel remorseful about missing her father's birthday because she is in the hospital. This in turn could lead to feelings of self-hate.
- Having a painful medical procedure. The experience of a stranger touching the patient could trigger feelings of fear and helplessness related to past trauma.
- Watching a violent film. This might cause the patient to recall and reexperience panic related to an assault he once suffered.
- A particular time of day (e.g., dusk) or time of year. For example, if a patient has lost loved ones around the holidays, she may feel increasing distress as this holiday period approaches and may want avoid the experience of the holiday or self-injure to relieve distress.

Events may trigger distress of greater magnitude than the nurse would expect. An understanding of a patient's discreet, individual triggers can help the patient and the nurse to anticipate when the additional levels of intervention are needed to manage the urge to self-injure. For a more in-depth discussion of this, please see Linehan, (1993).

Offer medication to prevent the onset of distress. Using the knowledge of identified triggers that cannot be avoided, the nurse and patient can arrange for the timely use of anxiolytic or other medication to reduce stress. For example, a prn medication might be offered before a family meeting or when the sun goes down.

● **Subgoal: Assist Patient in Learning and Using Alternative Coping Skills**

Assessment of Use of Alternative Coping Skills
In report. The nurse will want to know whether, in the last 24 hours, the patient has

- Shown increased understanding and/or acceptance of illness
- Voiced a desire to learn new skills
- Attended and participated in skills groups
- Asked the staff for help in using coping skills
- Used adaptive coping skills

One-to-one contact. During this time, the nurse will indirectly assess motivation to learn new coping skills by the way the patient speaks about her illness, hospitalization, and treatment. Is there evidence that the patient is taking responsibility for understanding difficulties and coming up with solutions? This patient may say, "I notice when I…." "today I learned…." Alternatively, does the patient use a language that suggests he is not ready for involvement in his own treatment, with phrases such as "you people" or "that doctor," or statements like "those groups are a waste of time"?

The nurse can also directly ask the patient about motivation to use or learn alternative (non-NSSI) coping skills. The nurse will ask what coping skills have been useful to this patient in the past and what kinds of coping skills might the patient might like to learn.

On the unit. The nurse will look for

- The patient's presence at and participation in groups as an indicator of willingness to learn new skills
- Any change in the patient's way of talking about illness with other patients as an indicator of willingness to take responsibility for one's own treatment

- The use of new coping skills: is the patient journaling or using the sensory room? Is he using sensory interventions such as headphones, holding frozen oranges in hands, the rocking chair, weighted blanket, or sour or hot candies?

● **Key Nursing Interventions to Increase the Use of Alternative Coping Skills**

Review treatment plan goals and review expectation of collaborative engagement. While meeting with patient, the nurse should explore patient goals for hospitalization and emphasize that collaboration between the patient and treatment team is essential for patient improvement. One way, the patient being a partner in his own treatment helps develop his own list of coping skills and form his own crisis plan. A crisis plan is simply a set of tasks the patient will employ to manage overwhelming feelings.

Help the patient to identify, learn, and use healthy coping skills. In the work with the treatment team, the patient will have identified some of the feelings, behaviors, thoughts, bodily sensations, events, or interactions that trigger distress. The nurse works to support the patient to learn and use coping skills when the patient feels distressed. Coping interventions can be in any of the eight following areas:

- Distress tolerance: activities that help manage emotional distress, self-destructive impulses, and other crises. For example, walking may help with distress tolerance. Initiating physical activity can have the benefit of changing the context of the distress, as well as activating endorphins. In addition, the patient might be reminded of other times when walking was pleasant or useful for tolerating distress.
- Self-Care: activities that take care of personal needs and physical health, such as taking a hot shower. These activ-

ities provide a change in context, as well as a physical sensation that grounds the person in the present.

- Mindfulness: intentionally focusing and giving complete attention to the one thing that the patient is doing in the present, noticing all aspects about it, without evaluating or judging the experience. For example, coloring can be an activity that draws a patient's focus to the present moment. The nurse will teach the patient that the very act of coloring is a coping skill and any resulting artwork is secondary.

- Sensory interventions: using the five senses to focus emotions and thoughts in the here and now. Examples include inhaling the aroma of lavender, sucking on sour candies, listening to soothing sounds, staring at a lava lamp or wearing colored glasses, squeezing a soft foam ball or a frozen orange, or sitting on a glider rocker under a weighted blanket. Any and all of these can shift the patient's experience by stimulating the senses and drawing attention to sensations in the moment.

- Cognitive restructuring: challenging negative thoughts and considering alternative ways to view a situation. This skill is often taught in groups.

- Affirmations: positive statements about oneself and one's ability to manage that helps build one's confidence and promote self-esteem. Affirmations can be taught in the groups on the milieu, or in the one-to-one contact. Examples of affirmations are "I am a good person," "I have skills and I can manage this situation," "I have raised three children so I can sort out this situation," and "I have felt this way before and it got better in a short time."

- Expression: communication of one's internal experience in a way that helps one to tolerate it and get support. Groups such as morning meeting and evening wrap-up group, therapy groups, and one-to-one contact offer opportunities for patients to express themselves and get support.

- Social connections: staying in contact with people in one's social support network and reaching out for help. The experience of a therapeutic milieu can teach a patient the skill of making contact. The nurse can also help her think about whom in her life can be part of a supportive network. The nurse can also encourage a patient to participate in available support and social groups after discharge.

Ideally, the patient develops an individualized coping skill list, and the nurse helps the patient use interventions from these areas to manage the distress he feels. This can complement the work that the patient does in groups. Once the nurses are familiar with the patient's plan, they can use it in every interaction with the patient, whether taking vital signs, administering meds, going on walks, or doing an assessment for the shift. Setting the expectation that the coping skills will help change the patient's experience will enhance success.

Identify and praise the use of alternative coping skills. The nurse will observe with the patient her efforts to use her crisis plan and validate with her the results of her efforts. Efforts by the patient are noted and communicated in report to the nursing staff and team, as well as to the patient. The nurse gives patient the positive feedbacks for the use of contracts, coping skills, or a crisis-prevention plan, regardless of outcome. In this way, the patient can begin to alter her view of herself from one of being helpless and a failure to one of being able to engage in slow progress.

Keep multiple copies of the coping skills and crisis prevention plan. The nurse will continue to refer to work being done on the coping skills and crisis-prevention plan by keeping a copy in the chart and making one for the patient to hold. Sometimes, in frustration, rage, or discouragement or to test the nurse's sincerity, a patient destroys what she has created. The nurse demonstrates his respect for the work by keeping an updated copy in the chart.

Encourage attendance at groups. It is in therapeutic milieu and therapy groups that staff teach coping skills.

Adopt a harm-reduction stance. When a patient has been unable to reduce the frequency of NSSI (e.g., she is still scratching her legs every night after visiting hours), the expectation of change may be too high, and so the nurse may offer a harm reduction plan. For example, the patient could rub her legs with ice or snap a rubber band instead of inducing more harmful NSSI.

TREATMENT ENGAGEMENT

● Subgoal: Increase Engagement in Treatment and Trust in Treatment Providers

Patients with self-injurious behavior may view hospitalization as an attempt to remove from them the main tool they have for coping with their distress. Therefore, patients may come feeling very mistrustful. Thus, building trust with the hospital, its staff, and the system is necessary before a patient can engage in treatment. Given the short lengths of stay for inpatient care in current times, there may not be significant engagement during the first or second hospitalization, but perhaps in a third or fourth hospitalization, there will be more.

Patients who use self-injurious behaviors as a coping skill are often those with enormous experience with relationships that have caused them great pain, and engaging in treatment may be a slow and difficult process. Patients must learn to trust a treatment provider enough to take a risk. Barent Walsh (Walsh, 2008) speaks of a gift, by which connections can sometimes be made in treatment that allows patients to take the risk of rethinking some of their core beliefs (negative, destructive and well ingrained). The gift is the therapeutic relationship through which a nurse or clinician conveys to patients that they have value, are lovable, and deserve to be well and unhurt. A gift is not easy to come by, but it is the compassion, consistency, and kindness of the nurse that makes such a connection a possibility. Then, many patients are able to consider letting go of old behaviors and begin to adopt adaptive coping strategies.

Assessment of Engagement in Treatment and Trust in Treatment Providers

In report, the nurse listens for

- History of a positive trusting relationship in the past
- Positive use of staff interventions
- Episodes of staff or unit splitting

one-to-one contact. During the one-to-one contact, the nurse assesses the patient's level of trust in her and in other staff. To do this, the nurse pays attention to the patient's

- Willingness to engage in conversation;
- Physical demeanor (body language, eye contact) that indicates how tense or relaxed the patient feels in the context of this interaction;
- Response to affirmations or challenges about the patient's work on the unit; and
- Ability to ask questions, challenge, or disagree with the nurse when necessary

On the unit, a patient's ability to use the groups safely and participate openly can be an indication of the ability to trust staff. However, sometimes, patients are most comfortable "running the show" and taking charge of the problems with the physical plant or another person's treatment rather than focusing on their own treatment. This may indicate some difficulty engaging in their work and trusting staff. In contrast, other patients may be quiet and not very visible on the unit, but working hard on their treatment.

● Key Nursing Interventions to Increase Engagement and Trust in Treatment Providers

Show non-judgmental compassion. The nurse will show empathy and will make efforts to be nonjudgmental. Although kindness is a treasured trait, patients who have had significant difficulty with relationships do not easily trust kindness or trust themselves to know what real kindness is. Walsh (2008, p. 77) describes something called "nonjudgmental compassion," which he contrasts with concern and support. The latter suggests an intense desire to protect and intervene. This is a problem because the nurse takes on the responsibility for the NSSI; this responsibility in fact belongs to the patient. Instead, the nurse should strive for nonjudgmental compassion, which is related to *acceptance.* The nurse will try to show acceptance for the patient as a person, regardless of the symptoms and troublesome behaviors the patient may bring with him onto the unit. The nurse does this by letting the patient know that she *values the patient even when he uses NSSI,* using emotional nonresponse when necessary, and maintaining consistency.

Use good communication skills. The nurse will state expectations and consequences clearly, give honest feedback, and validate the patient's experience. This shows respect for the patient and provides an example of how to communicate clearly. Clear communication may not be common in the patient's other relationships.

Give the patient the opportunity to grow and change. The nurse will acknowledge the patient's growth and progress during the hospitalization. For instance, the nurse will advocate for decreasing safety orders, so the patient who has demonstrated readiness can shave unsupervised or use the hair dryer independently.

Be consistent. All of these interventions will assist the patient with the experience of a trusting relationship with staff, consistency, especially when it seems contrary to the patient's expressed wish, is the most important. Consistency helps the patient know what to expect, so she can take charge of her own behavior. The patient will know, for instance, that self-injury will result in the need for remaining in open areas, or a loss of privileges, rather than an increase in one-to-one time. If the consequences are not consistent, the patient will not always know what to expect. This creates enormous anxiety for the patient and likely replicates some previous negative experiences of an uncertain world with traumatic results.

Understand that building trust is difficult for the patient and takes time. The nurse should keep in mind that she cannot force a trusting relationship to happen. Instead, the nurse should provide an opportunity for the patient to have a new relationship experience. The nurse then hopes that the patient can take this experience of compassion, consistency, and honesty, along with his new coping skills, with him when he leaves the hospital.

As the patient practices a trusting relationship, he may test the limits of this relationship. Often, this is referred to as "gaminess" and seen as insincere behavior. For example, a patient may agree to tell the nurse about urges to cut, while at the same time cutting and hiding the implement and the cuts. In response, the nurse needs to consistently implement the treatment plan and accept that this is the best the patient can do right now. The nurse's own feelings of disappointment, anger, and betrayal should be shared separately with a supervisor or colleague, while the patient is offered nonjudgmental compassion.

PREPARATION FOR DISCHARGE

Patients with NSSI are often discharged quickly because they do not meet current level of care criteria for inpatient care. Most often, this criterion is that the patient is a danger to herself or others by virtue of mental illness. While this patient may engage in self-harm, she may not have any suicidal ideation. Thus, there may be no compelling need for inpatient level of care. Some will need and qualify for residential treatment where they can continue to learn ways to manage overwhelming emotions.

Preparation for discharge will include a patient's preparation of a comprehensive, personalized coping skills list, a plan for acquiring the things he will need to cope (e.g., ranging from a support group to a lavender scented candle), and a detailed aftercare treatment plan. Often, patients with NSSI will revert to self-injurious behavior as the time of discharge nears. The nurse needs to understand this behavior as a sign of increased anxiety. The nurse can anticipate this and assist the patient by telling the patient that he expects that the patient will feel increased anxiety as discharge nears. The nurse may then go on to explore of fears associated with discharge and the return to the community. The nurse's acceptance of these fears helps to make the patient feel that these fears are both normal and manageable.

TABLE 5.1
Goals, Areas of Assessment, and Interventions for a Patient With Nonsuicidal Self-Injury

Goal	Assessment	Intervention
	Safety	
Prevent unintentional lethality from NSSI	Gather information about recent suicidal thoughts and behaviors and risky NSSI behavior Assess whether any serious and stressful life events have recently occurred Ask about ambivalence about living Understand history of suicidality Look for increases in medical severity of self-harm Assess environmental safety Watch for increases in patient's level of agitation or secretive or isolative behaviors	Increase level of observation Explore ambivalence and understand impulsivity Ensure environmental safety on the unit Use restraint as a last resort
Reduce frequency and severity of NSSI	Assess frequency and severity of urges to self-injure and actual NSSI Look for episodes of anxiety or agitation and assess which interventions are helpful for these episodes Assess whether the patient believes NSSI is a problem Watch for changes in patient behavior	Negotiate an agreement that the patient will inform staff if she feels at risk of self-harm Offer prn medication Utilize sensory interventions Have a plan for what will happen should the patient engage in self-harm Establish an appropriate level of supervision Employ room changes Note and acknowledge any decreased frequency or severity of NSSI

(cont.)

TABLE 5.1
Goals, Areas of Assessment, and Interventions for a Patient With Nonsuicidal Self-Injury   (cont.)

Goal	Assessment	Intervention
	Stabilization	
Identify and decrease the distress that is an antecedent of NSSI	Note any episodes of distress and look for precipitating events or triggers Assess whether the patient has an increased capacity to name feelings	Help patients identify emotions that may trigger impulses for NSSI Validate the patient's feelings Remind the patient that feelings cannot be avoided but can be managed Help patients identify other triggers for urges to self-injure Offer medication to prevent the onset of distress
Assist patient in learning and using alternative coping skills	Assess patient's willingness to learn new coping skills Look for use of new coping skills	Review treatment plan goals and review expectation of collaborative engagement Help the patient to identify, learn, and use healthy coping skills Identify and praise the use of alternative coping skills Keep multiple copies of the coping skills and crisis prevention plan Encourage attendance at groups Adopt a harm-reduction stance

(cont.)

TABLE 5.1
Goals, Areas of Assessment, and Interventions for a Patient With
Nonsuicidal Self-Injury (cont.)

Goal	Assessment	Intervention
Treatment Engagement		
Increase engagement in treatment and trust in treatment providers	Assess the patient's degree of trust in the nurse and other treatment providers Look for a willingness to engage in conversation and to respond to staff comments or concerns	Show nonjudgmental compassion Use good communication skills Give the patient an opportunity to grow and change Be consistent Understand that building trust is difficult for the patient and takes time
Subgoal: assist patient with the experience of a trusting relationship	Assess for a history of a positive trusting relationship in the past; positive use of staff interventions; episodes of staff or unit splitting	The nurse continues to respond with: consistency, empathy, neutrality (non judgmental), clear expectations, clearly stated consequences, honest feedback, and supportive validation

REFERENCES

Beck, J. (2005). *Cognitive therapy for challenging problems.* New York: Guilford Press.

Comtois, K. A. (2002). A review of interventions to reduce the prevalence of parasuicide. *Psychiatric Services, 53,* 1138–1144.

Hawton, K., Townsend, E., Arensman, E., Gunnell, D., Hazell, P., House, A., & vanHeeringen, K. (2000). Psychosocial versus pharmacological treatments for deliberate self-harm. *Cochrane Database of Systematic Reviews, 2,* CD 001764.

Hicks, K. M., & Hinck, S. M. (2008). Concept analysis of self-mutilation. *Journal of Advanced Nursing, 64,* 408–413.

Kalafat, J., & Lester, D. (2000). Shame and suicide: A case study. *Death Studies, 24,* 157–162.

Knight, M., Adkison, L., Kovach, J. (2010). A comparison of multisensory and traditional interventions on inpatient psychiatry and geriatric neuropsychiatry units. *Journal of Psychosocial Nursing & Mental Health Services, 48,* 1: 24031.

Linehan, M. M. (1993). *Skills training manual for treating borderline personality disorder.* New York: Guilford Press.

Nock, M. K. (2009). Why do people hurt themselves? New insights into the nature and functions of self-injury. *Current Directions in Psychological Science, 18,* 78–83.

Shea, S. (1999). *The practical art of suicide assessment: A guide for mental health professionals and substance abuse counselors.* New York: Wiley.

Simeon, D., & Favazza A. (2001). Self-injurious behavior behaviors, phenomenology and assessment. In D. Simeon, & E. Hollander (Eds.), *Self-injurious behaviors, assessment and treatment* (pp. 1–29). Washington, DC: American Psychiatric Association.

Van Sell, S. L., O'Quin, L., Oliphant, E., Shull, P., Austin, K., Johnston, E., & Nguyen, C. (2005), Self-injury. *RN, 68,* 55–58.

Walsh, B. W. (2008). *Treating self injury: A practical guide.* New York: Guilford Press.

Young, R., Sweeting, H., & West, P. (2006), Prevalence of deliberate self harm and attempted suicide within contemporary Goth youth subculture: Longitudinal cohort study. *British Medical Journal, 332,* 1058–1061.

The Patient in Pain

6

Ellen Blair, Karen Larsen, and Cynthia Belonick

BACKGROUND AND DESCRIPTION

Pain is defined as an "unpleasant sensory and emotional experience arising from actual or potential tissue damage or described in terms of such damage." It can have a sudden or slow onset of any intensity from mild to severe (International Association of the Study of Pain [IASP], 2010). Pain can be acute and associated with a recent onset of injury or tissue damage. Pain may diminish as healing occurs. It can also be chronic with a persistent presence for 6 months or more, and lasting beyond when healing would have been expected. Pain is a unique subjective state whereby the patient may experience a wide range of unpleasant sensations and distress. Physical pain is usually considered *neuropathic, somatic,* or *visceral* in origin. Neuropathic pain can result from injury or dysfunction to the peripheral or central nervous system; somatic pain originates from nociceptive receptor activation in the skin, subcutaneous tissue, bone, muscle, or blood vessels. Nociceptive receptors are sensory nerve endings that can detect mechanical, thermal, or chemical changes above a set threshold. Once stimulated, a nociceptor transmits a signal along the spinal cord to the brain. Visceral pain also originates from nociceptive activation, but in the internal organs.

In clinical practice, pain can be defined as whatever the experiencing person says it is, and existing whenever she says it does. Extensive studies of the anatomy, physiology, and pharmacology show that the perceived intensity of pain is not proportional to the type or extent of tissue damage (Massie, 2000; IASP, 2010).

Until the mid 1960s, the predominant view was a biomedical model of pain; that is, pain was considered a symptom of underlying disease or tissue damage, and successful treatment of the disease or damage should lead to resolution of the pain. Melzack and Wall (1965) introduced the gate control theory of pain in an article in *Science* entitled "Pain Mechanisms: A New Theory." Unlike the biomedical model, the gate control theory suggested that pain perception is a complex phenomenon, and the experience and physiology of pain are not only the result of tissue damage or disease on the periphery, but were also affected by emotional and cognitive states that can modify the pain experience.

The gate control theory states that pain is transmitted through a process typically beginning in the periphery, although, as already described, it can also begin in the central nervous system or internal organs. Transduction of pain stimuli begins at the time of the injury or tissue damage. The dorsal horn area in the spinal cord works like a gate to increase or decrease the painful messages through the spinal cord and to the brain. Conscious perception of pain occurs when there is transmission from the spinal cord to the brain.

In addition to actual tissue damage or injury, the individual's emotional or past traumatic life experiences may intensify the opening of the pain "gate," whereas the direction of attention away from the pain may actually close the pain "gate." When the patient has onset of pain at an early age or chronic pain, such as failed back syndrome, phantom limb pain, and reflex sympathetic dystrophy, changes may occur in the nervous system itself, which not only alter how pain is perceived and processed but also cause both hypersensitivity and hyperalgesia. As a result, the patient's pain threshold, the point where pain begins to be felt for that particular person, is lowered (Gatchel & Turk, 1999). For these individuals, the pain gate can be easily opened. Because the pain threshold may be altered in the central nervous system, these patients may have difficulty coping with pain affecting other bodily systems as well (i.e., cardiovascular, endocrine, pulmonary, and gastrointestinal).

Modulation of pain occurs when there is a release of endorphins, serotonin, and epinephrine in the brain, thus inhibiting the pain impulse from being communicated to the next neuron. This may "close the gate" and decrease the pain perception. A simple example illustrates this: If someone bumps her knee, a message is sent to the brain and she may start rubbing her knee. This stimulates fibers to release endorphins. By doing so, the pain impulses are altered, therefore changing the perception of pain (closing the gate) and diminishing the pain (St. Marie, 2002).

Behavior

The patient in pain, preoccupied with self and the pain experience, may exhibit social withdrawal and isolation. Facial grimacing, verbal expression of pain, crying, pacing, restlessness, and rocking may also be behavioral manifestations. Guarding the affected area of the body; slow, difficult movement; and/or rigid positioning and posturing are common. Pain, as well as the anticipation of pain, can cause severe stress, decreasing a person's strength, coordination, and independence. Moreover, the patient in pain may avoid certain situations to prevent the pain from recurring. Avoidant behavior can be maladaptive if the patient begins to avoid important daily activities, responsibilities related to work, or relationships with others. In addition, patients may become hostile and reject well-meaning assistance while still appearing needy and unable to adequately care for themselves (Leo, 2003).

A patient's culture, race, ethnicity, financial or religious background, and drug history can influence his or her behavioral response to pain and willingness to accept care (Leo, 2003). We provide some examples here; however, it is important to note that there are substantial individual differences in pain expression within every cultural group. Some people from cultures that value stoicism (such as the Chinese culture) may not moan, scream, or even grimace when in pain. They may strive to keep their faces "masked." Feeling that they will be perceived as weak if they admit to pain, they may even deny having pain when asked. They may prefer to be left alone to bear their pain without bothering others and may have learned to cope without seeking attention or care (Lasch, 2000). It is important for the nurse to be aware that common beliefs regarding cultural groups can result in mismanagement. For example, Native Americans are often viewed as stoic and able to bear much pain. This view, combined with the stereotype that they are prone to substance abuse, may lead to undertreatment of pain (Narayan, 2010).

Other cultural groups, such as Italians, Arabians, and African Americans, may be more expressive about pain. Individuals from these groups may be taught in childhood that when one is in pain, the appropriate or best response is to moan, cry, groan, or scream. Some groups encourage individuals in pain to seek attention and support and encourage caregivers to attend to them. Contrary to the more stoic cultural characteristics, members of these groups may prefer not to be alone when they are in pain (Narayan, 2010).

Cognition

Psychological and emotional processes affect perceptions of pain. It is important to understand the meaning of pain and suffering, and how the patient interprets the impact of her pain on quality of life, that is, the ability to work, fulfill responsibilities, be part of a family, and form close relationships. Beliefs about pain can help or hinder successful coping, and can be associated with distress or, conversely, hopefulness. Types of maladaptive ways of thinking about pain may include catastrophizing, helplessness, magnification, personalization, and self-fulfilling prophecies (Adams, Poole, & Richardson, 2006; Leo, 2003).

Catastrophizing involves a belief that one's situation can only get worse and that all is lost. The patient may say, "I will always have this pain, and therefore I will always be miserable." Helplessness is the belief that nothing that one does matters or can provide relief. The patient may say, "My doctor says that if I exercise, the pain will get better, but I know it will not help!" Magnification is the exaggeration of the significance of a negative event. The patient may relate the pain to work. For example, a patient might say, "My pain got worse at work yesterday, and I had to leave early. I might as well accept that I am totally disabled." Personalization directly relates an event or a problem to oneself or one's limitations. The patient may say, "I am being punished for all the mistakes in my life— this pain is all my fault." Self-fulfilling prophecies occur when one expects adverse outcomes and then contributes to life scenarios to fulfill these expectations. For example, the patient who anticipates that his spouse will reject him becomes short tempered. This may lead the spouse to withdraw and avoid her husband, thus confirming the patient's expectations and creating a cycle of maladaptive behaviors (Leo, 2003).

Pain can alter the patient's self-perception and raise fears of being isolated or misunderstood. For example, a patient may believe she is less interesting and desirable to others, is weak, immature, dirty, or contagious (Massie, 2000). It is common for patients in pain to harbor certain fears: fear of addiction, fear of being labeled "a complainer" or "med seeking," and ultimately the fear of losing control. Finally, in the case of pain associated with terminal illness, thoughts about death and dying typically arise.

Affect

Pain often includes unpleasant emotions such as anxiety or sadness (Gatchel & Turk, 1999). Individuals may worry about the future or mourn past losses, including losses of functioning related to the pain. Persistent symptoms, an inconclusive diagnosis, or repeated treatment failures creates anxiety, frustration, or anger toward the health care system, employer, family members, or oneself. Irritability or hostility can often mask the underlying fear and sadness.

Context

Physical malady and mental illness often coexist (Gatchel, 2004b). Pain is frequently comorbid with or part of psychiatric diagnoses including, but not limited to, somatoform disorder, hypochondriasis, posttraumatic stress disorder, psychotic disorders, organic brain diseases (including types of dementias), substance abuse, depression, and anxiety (American Psychiatric Association [APA], 2000; Dewar, 2009; Townsend, 2006). Although this is not an all-inclusive list, the wide variety of conditions reinforces the need to conduct a pain assessment on each hospitalized psychiatric patient, at least once a shift. In fact, in most hospitals, pain is considered the "fifth vital sign," and therefore an important indicator of the patient's overall health status (APA, 2000; Dewar et al., 2009; Townsend, 2006).

POTENTIAL BARRIERS TO BEING THERAPEUTIC

Concerns about legitimacy of a patient's pain. The nurse's own experience with pain and beliefs about pain; the nurse's conversations with the patient, family, nurses, and other health care providers; the perceived source of pain in the patient; the presence of other psychiatric diagnoses (including Axis II diagnoses) in the patient; and the general environment of the treatment team on the inpatient unit can all significantly affect the way the nurse perceives and responds to the patient experiencing pain. In some cases, the nurse may believe that the patient is (consciously or unconsciously) lying or exaggerating her degree of pain to obtain, among other things, more medication. If the nurse doubts the legitimacy of the patient's pain, this may evoke anger, frustration, resentment, and a lack of empathy on the part of the nurse. These feelings can be in conflict with the nurse's identity as a helpful, caring, and nurturing individual. The nurse's perceptions of the legitimacy of pain can also be a key factor in choosing to administer PRN analgesics (Dewar et al., 2009). If, for example, a patient was in a car accident prior to admission, the nurse will more likely consider the pain legitimate and may readily decide to offer or administer analgesics. However, when there is no known or obvious etiology of pain or when there is a history of substance abuse, the nurse may feel frustrated or helpless in her ability to assess validity of the pain and may choose not to administer an analgesic when it is requested (Dewar et al., 2009).

Caring for the addicted patient who is experiencing pain can be particularly challenging. Again, the "legitimacy" of the pain may be questioned. A nurse can easily assume that the patient requesting a pain medication is "drug seeking" and lying or exaggerating his degree of pain to obtain more medication. Although many addicted patients resolve their discomfort by seeking a substance, this does not mean that the addicted patient's pain is not real. Moreover, an addicted patient may legitimately have a need for more pain medications compared with a person of equal size. Long-standing exposure to foreign substances, as with addictions, accelerates enzyme systems, thus deactivating any medication more swiftly. Therefore, in addition to the psychological need to have more pain relief through higher doses of pain meds and more frequent dosing, there is also a physiological reason for "med-seeking behavior."

In these cases, it is important that the nurse return to the fact that the person expressing physical pain is in very real distress and that the patient needs to communicate that distress. The nurse must find ways to respect the patient's experience so that he can be truly present for the patient and adequately address problems with physical pain.

OVERVIEW OF NURSING CARE GOALS

1. Safety
   - Prevent or reduce the risk for harm to self
2. Stabilization
   - Reduce or alleviate pain symptoms
   - Decrease the patient's pain-related anxiety
   - Help the patient to improve functioning in the presence of pain
3. Engagement
   - Engage the patient in treatment despite the experience of pain

---

Although a chronic physical illness and its symptoms may not be viewed as a priority during an acute inpatient psychiatric hospitalization, the presence of pain must be treated as "real" (not simply as part of a particular personality style) and "relevant" (not something to be dealt with after discharge). Dismissing the pain ignores a critical problem that contributes to physical, mental, and spiritual anguish.

SAFETY

● Subgoal: Prevent or Reduce the Risk for Harm to Self

This section will review suicide assessment as it pertains specifically to the patient with physical pain; however, please refer to Chapter 9, "The Patient Who Is Suicidal," for more in-depth information on suicide assessment and intervention.

Patients with chronic pain have high rates of attempted or completed suicides. In fact, the prevalence of suicide in the population with pain is estimated to be twice that of groups without pain (St. Marie, 2002; Tang & Crane, 2006). Factors associated with pain, such as poor sleep and disruptions in work, family activities, or independence, can result in financial stressors, legal complications, isolation, and hopelessness. Depression can ensue, leaving the patient with a desperate need to escape, either through substance abuse or through suicide. A patient in pain and with a comorbid substance abuse problem has an increased risk for completed suicide (St. Marie, 2002). In addition, the presence of back pain or widespread body pain is associated with a higher risk of future death by suicide. Finally, longer pain duration is associated with increased likelihood of suicidal ideation (Tang & Crane, 2006).

Pain from cancer is among the most significant contributors to emotional distress. Helplessness, hopelessness, and irritability engendered by unrelieved pain foster fears of being unable to cope, particularly at the end of life. Anxiety reactions, fears of a loss of control, phobias, and panic attacks can ensue. Thus, cancer patients with severe, unrelieved pain are more likely to consider and to commit suicide than other pain populations (Lancee et al., 1994; Massie & Holland, 1990; Tang & Crane, 2006).

Assessment of Risk for Harm to Self
In report. Nurses and other staff must communicate risk factors for suicide, including hopelessness; helplessness; isolation; change in affect, mood, energy, eating, and sleeping patterns; having access to weapons; and any recent stressful events, including discouraging medical news. Other risk factors the nurse should note are the patient's history of suicide, positive family history of suicide, location

and duration of pain (as noted previously, the presence of back pain or allover body pain, or a longer duration of pain, is associated with increased suicidality or thoughts of self-harm), and comorbid depression (Tang & Crane, 2006).

One-to-one contact. During the individual contact, the nurse will convey nonjudgmental and empathetic style. She should ask the patient about how he is feeling and then directly ask, "Have you thought about harming yourself in any way, or even taking your own life? If so, what do you plan to do? Sometimes when people experience such terrible pain, they become very hopeless and may not even want to go on with their lives. I understand." Particularly relevant are questions to determine whether helplessness or hopelessness related to controlling pain is associated with suicidal thoughts. For example, a patient may say, "I feel like I have nothing left to live for; nothing is going to help my pain, and I will not be able to do anything that I used to care about."

On the unit. Depending on the level of suicidality, the nurse should provide an appropriate level of observation. A patient who is receiving medication for pain, such as opiates, antianxiety agents, and/or sleeping medications, should be closely monitored to be sure he is truly taking the medication and not "cheeking" or "mouthing" the medication (securing the medication under the tongue or tucked into the inner mouth cheek) to be stockpiled and hoarded for a future overdose. Drug overdose is the most common method of suicide among patients with chronic pain, especially in those who have survived a previous suicide attempt (Tang & Crane, 2006).

● Key Nursing Interventions to Reduce the Risk of Harm to Self

Create a safe environment for the patient. The nurse should remove all potentially harmful objects that the patient can access, including belts, sharp objects, straps, ties, glass items, and lighters. Searching the room may also be necessary. Due to the risk of mouthing or cheeking medications, supervision during meals and medication administration are important. If there is suspicion that the patient is not taking her medication, the nurse may wish to institute a mouth-check process at medication time, based on the institution's specific policy.

Discourage isolation. Patients in pain may have a tendency to isolate. Because suicide risk may decrease when a patient feels connected to others, a patient found isolating should be encouraged to attend unit activities and groups and spend time with others. Out-of-room activities as simple as sitting in the dayroom can help the patient to feel less alone and less focused on physical pain and its accompanying negative thoughts or thoughts of hopelessness—even if only for a brief period of time (Gatchel, 2004b; Townsend, 2006).

Express realistic hope about the future. Talking with the patient about coping mechanisms that worked well in the past and strengths that can support him in the present and future can be most helpful. The nurse should provide expressions of hope to the patient in a positive, low-key manner. For example, the nurse might say, "I know you feel you cannot go on with this amount of pain, but we are hoping to *buy some time* so we can work together to make life, once again, worth living. You've found solace in attending religious services in the past; I'm hoping you will find that helpful once again." The nurse can express hope that although the pain may never go away entirely, there may be strategies—medical or other—that the patient has not tried that could better manage the pain or the person's ability to cope with pain. The nurse should avoid absolutes such as "I know we'll find something that makes your pain go away" or "Your pain is only temporary—it won't last forever." Statements like these offer false hope to the patient, are often not believable, and may undermine trust.

Treat the physical pain. Since the pain causes human anguish and contributes to feelings of suicidality, hopelessness, and depression, treating pain will be critical. By treating and managing the patient's painful symptoms, the nurse communicates that the pain is real. This can feel very validating to a patient who may not have gotten this message from other health care providers or family members.

STABILIZATION

● **Subgoal: Reduce or Alleviate Pain Symptoms**

Assessment of Pain Intensity and Severity
Basic principles in conducting a pain assessment include

- Assessing pain on a regular basis;
- Soliciting the patient's self-report of the pain experience if possible;
- Accepting the patient's self-report;
- Using a single-rating scale over time as an index of pain severity; and
- Tracking and documenting pain severity scores and other aspects of the pain experience (St. Marie, 2002).

In report. A proactive assessment of pain begins during report. When hearing that a patient is in pain, the nurse should ask and/or consider the following questions: Where is the pain? How does the patient describe the pain? How long has the patient had the pain? Has there been a thorough medical evaluation of the etiology of the pain? How is the patient coping? Is pain the chief complaint for admission to the hospital? What helps reduce or eliminate the pain? How does the patient's cultural or other background potentially inform how she is expressing and coping with the pain? Answers to these questions will provide information about additional assessments needed and how to choose interventions for an individualized care plan.

One-to-one contact. During the initial and subsequent meetings with the patient, the nurse will perform a thorough pain assessment to understand the patient's pain experience.

First, the nurse will look for nonverbal symptoms of pain, such as facial grimacing, guarding, or protecting the part of the body experiencing pain, tearful or anxious behaviors, pacing, restlessness, and rocking. Second, because there can be an autonomic response from pain, the nurse will check the patient's vital signs, reporting any changes/abnormalities from baseline measurements to the treatment team. The nurse will also assess for diaphoreses, pupil dilatation, pallor, and nausea. Third, because a patient in pain can experience an altered perception of time, the nurse should assess orientation to date, time, and place. Fourth, the nurse will ask the patient questions about the pain. He will want to ask about the location and quality of the pain. With regard to location of pain, the nurse should be aware of the concept of "referred pain," that is, pain that presents in an area removed or distant from its point of origin (St. Marie, 2002). Examples of referred pain are back pain that is actually caused by a disease of the pancreas or upper back, and chest and arm pain (even pain in the ear or jaw) that actually signals a heart attack. With regard to the quality of pain, words that the patient uses may provide information about diagnosis or useful treatments. "Sore" or "achy" may indicate somatic pain that may respond well to nonsteroidal anti-inflammatory drugs (NSAIDs) or heat or cold. "Burning" or "electric" suggest neuropathic pain that may respond well to anticonvulsants or tricyclic antidepressants (Leo, 2003; Massie, 2000; Townsend, 2006).

The nurse will ask about the onset and duration of the pain: "Was the onset gradual or sudden?" "Is the duration of the pain intermittent or persistent?" "Is there break-through pain?" She will ask whether there are there any factors that precipitate the pain. The nurse will assess the patient's knowledge of and preference for pain-relieving strategies and the patient's expectations regarding pain relief. The nurse will also look for and ask about side effects of medications (such as sedation) along with the effectiveness of both medications and nonpharmacologic therapies.

Finally, the nurse will ask the patient to rate current pain using the pain severity scale used in the hospital. (The most popular is the severity scale of 0 to 10, with 0 being no pain and 10 being the worst pain imaginable.) A pain severity scale is important because it provides an easy and consistent way to track changes over time and therefore may be used to assess the effectiveness of different pain-relieving strategies. Also, such a scale may provide a more "universal" approach to the assessment of pain by transcending some of individual or cultural differences in expressing, describing, and reporting pain.

Patients with cognitive impairment, such as patients with dementia, psychotic symptoms, or vegetative depression, may be unable to report pain symptoms. These patients are particularly vulnerable to undertreatment for pain (Dewar, 2009). Hence, attention to nonverbal manifestations of pain is paramount. Potential structured tools to use when patients cannot self-report are the Non-Communicative Patient's Pain Assessment Instrument (Horgas, Nichols, Schapson, & Vietes, 2007) and the Behavioral Pain Scale for Intubated Patients (Payen, 2001). If these scales are not available, the nurse should objectively assess the patient for pain based on the following behaviors:

- *Negative vocalization*: moaning, screaming, crying out, grunting, whimpering, swearing, name-calling, weeping;

- *Facial expression*: sad, frightened, frown, wincing, grimacing, clenched teeth, quivering chin;
- *Body position*: rigid, tense, knees drawn up;
- *Body movement*: fidgeting, squirming, rocking, restless, rubbing of a body part, pulling away when touched;
- *Noisy breathing*: rapid breathing, hyperventilation, sighing;
- *Decreased function*: difficulty sleeping, refusal to eat or drink, resisting attempts to move or mobilize; and
- *Vital signs*: all changes should raise suspicion.

On the unit. The nurse should watch for the pain-related behaviors described above, and note consistencies, or inconsistencies, between self-reports and behaviors. It is not likely that a patient with pain at a "10" on the pain severity scale will be able to read a book. Patients with severe pain often do not appear rested. Although the nurse may see pain in their facial expressions, this is not always the case. Furthermore, the patient in pain may withdraw from social or physical contact. Self-absorption contributes to this isolation. The patient in pain may lose connections to the outside world, may become less verbal, less interested in current events, and even disinterested in visitors. If the nurse sees isolative behaviors, he will try to discern whether it is related to pain, psychiatric or medical problem, or some combination of problems.

● **Key Nursing Interventions for Reducing or Alleviating Pain Symptoms**

Assist the physician with finding the source of the pain and selecting effective interventions. The nurse's observations can provide essential information that may help the physician with diagnosis of the cause of pain or choice of best pain-management strategies. In addition to the pain assessment on each shift, the nurse should monitor laboratory results for physiological changes that may support underlying disease processes and review interdisciplinary assessments. This will give the nurse a comprehensive picture of the patient's pain experience; she should then communicate information about pain in shift report/handoff and in her documentation. It is particularly important for the nurse to work closely with the prescriber when the pain is unrelieved or the etiology of the pain is undetermined.

Administer medication to reduce or alleviate pain. Administering medications, specifically analgesics, is an important part of the nurse's role in pain management. Knowledge about the medications being administered, including potential side effects, is critical. There are many different types of analgesics. The most common types used in the inpatient psychiatric setting are NSAIDs (e.g., ibuprofen and naproxen), and opioids (e.g., oxycodone, methadone, and tramadol). Opioids can be considered "mild" (e.g., codeine) or "strong" (e.g., morphine, oxycodone, and methadone). Adjuvant medications are often used in conjunction with analgesics to achieve optimal patient comfort and symptom-specific pain relief. These adjuvant medications include anti-inflammatories, muscle relaxers, anti-anxiety medications, corticosteroids, antidepressants, anticonvulsants, topical medications, and sleep aids.

There are objective and formal guidelines for administering pain medication. A useful general practice guideline is the World Health Organization's "three-step analgesic ladder," which is a hierarchy of prescription medication progression in the treatment of pain (St. Marie, 2002). Although originally designed for cancer pain, it is also useful for noncancer pain. If pain occurs,

- Promptly administer nonopioids (aspirin and acetaminophen) orally with or without adjuvant medications;
- Then, as necessary, administer mild opioids (codeine) with or without adjuvant medications; and

- Finally, if the patient continues to experience pain, administer strong opioids with or without nonopioids and adjuvant medications

Many physicians will follow some version of these guidelines as they select treatments. Other information that may contribute to the physician's development of an individualized regime of pain medication includes the patient's physiology, symptoms, and past response to pharmacological treatments.

The most frequently used options for dosing of pain medications are "around-the-clock" (ATC) dosing or "prn" (i.e., "as needed") dosing. Though different, their use should be geared toward similar goals: to prevent the pain from recurring, to reduce the patient's anxiety over the thought of the pain returning, and to reduce the total dose of medication used to manage the pain. Whatever option of dosing is selected, the nurse should be familiar with the term "getting on top of the pain." This term refers to medicating the patient at the earliest stage of discomfort, that is, before the pain becomes overwhelming. If this is not done, the medication will take significantly longer period to produce a satisfactory response. For patients with continuous pain who continue to also need frequent prn dosing for pain relief, the physician will often transition the patient to a long-acting opioid as an ATC medication with a prn dose allowed for breakthrough pain.

Intermittent or prn dosing is appropriate when the pain is episodic or when "rescue" doses are needed in addition to a continuous dose schedule for breakthrough pain. Fast-acting opioids (e.g., morphine, oxycodone, hydromorphone, and codeine) are the medications of choice for prn dosing because they are effective for short periods of time (St. Marie, 2002). Medicating as needed (i.e., prn) requires the nurse to critically think about how and when to medicate while also assessing the patient for any adverse side effects prior to administering the medication.

Factors the nurse might think about include "Is the patient asking for medication?" "When was the last time the medication was given?" "Could the ATC dose be inadequate?" or "Are there any nonmedication interventions that might relieve pain?"

Regardless of the type of analgesic medication and dosing schedule, once an analgesic is given, the nurse should document the effect (usually by asking the patient to provide a pain rating on the 10-point pain-severity scale) within an hour post administration so the patient's response can be evaluated against the expected outcome, and more aggressive measures can be instituted as needed. At the same time, the nurse should also watch for possible untoward side effects of the pain medication, such as excessive sedation, unsteadiness, complaints of dizziness, or confusion. Any of these side effects should be communicated to the prescriber and treatment team immediately, as these are not only uncomfortable for the patient but can also put the patient at risk for falling. If these side effects are noted, the nurse might consider holding the medication pending further assessment and collaboration with the team.

The prescription of opioid medications for pain can be controversial. Opioids are addictive and can have adverse side effects such as constipation, excessive sedation, respiratory depression, and, in some cases, even death. Opioids can also be misused or diverted. On the other hand, it is also critically important to treat pain adequately, and opioids can be an important tool in the medication arsenal. Some physicians use the Screener and Opioid Assessment for Patients with Pain (Webster & Dove, 2007) as a tool to assess and screen patients for the use of long-term opioid therapy. This tool aids in identifying patients who may have some maladaptive behaviors and therefore require more treatment boundaries and vigilance on the part of the practitioner. We discuss more about the nurse's feelings about providing opioids in Chapter 17, "Management of Barriers to Being Therapeutic."

Along with monitoring medications for pain and the patient's response, the psychiatric nurse may be called upon to oversee a "medication reduction" program in the inpatient psychiatric setting. Many patients with pain become over-reliant on pain-relief medications and may combine pain medications with over-the-counter medications, alcohol, and illegal substances. The result can be a dangerous drug–drug interaction, toxicity, or death. Once hospitalized, every effort must be made to prevent severe withdrawal reactions. A structured, medically supervised detoxification protocol often becomes a component of a chronic pain management program. This protocol, which is discussed with the patient in advance, typically includes a medication reduction plan where the dose of medication is systematically and gradually reduced. During the "tapering regimen," the nurse will support the patient to find effective nonpharmacological coping strategies to replace chemical use and abuse (Simon, 1996).

Teach about medications. The nurse will educate patients about pain medications (as well as all prescribed psychiatric medications) and the importance of taking these as prescribed. Key topics to cover include dosing and timing regimen, side effects of medication, safe storage of the medication(s), and when to report inadequate pain relief or concerning side effects. The nurse will also instruct the patient that he should not change the amount or frequency of the medication without discussing it with his provider. Since the patient experiencing pain may have difficulty concentrating, the nurse should also suggest the patient to keep a calendar for medication scheduling and use a medication box to organize his medications, especially if the patient takes several medications. With the patient's consent, the nurse should also give the family and significant caregivers the instructions for medication administration to help ensure the best retention of information.

Teach the patient how to accurately report her pain. Pain education includes teaching the patient to discern and accurately report location, duration, intensity, and alleviating or aggravating factors. Instructing the patient to evaluate and report effectiveness of treatment helps create a realistic plan of care. To offer the patient more control and to learn more about his pain symptoms, the nurse can suggest the patient keep a "pain diary," or journal of his pain symptoms, recording variables such as time of day pain occurs and types of activities that worsen or improve the pain.

The nurse may want to familiarize the patient with the gate control theory of pain (described earlier in this chapter), the term "pain threshold," and the many factors that contribute to the experience of pain. By increasing the patient's knowledge about how she can increase the threshold for pain, and the ways the pain experience can be altered, the nurse is offering the patient a mechanism to increase control over what is typically viewed as an uncontrollable situation.

Teach relaxation and distraction techniques. Relaxation techniques can augment other strategies for pain relief. The goal is to reduce muscle tension, which subsequently reduces pain (particularly musculoskeletal pain) and anxiety. Relaxation therapies include progressive muscle relaxation, deep breathing exercises, biofeedback, guided imagery, meditation, music therapy, and even humor. (Please see Chapter 13, "Relaxation Techniques," for more information.) Distraction techniques heighten a person's concentration on a nonpainful activity and decrease the awareness and experience of pain. Involving the patient in a favorite activity, such as playing a card game with a visitor, listening to music, or playing with an electronic handheld game, can be an effective psychological intervention. The more involved the patient becomes in the activity, the greater the distraction from the pain.

Provide nursing comfort measures. Interventions that can be used in or out of the hospital may include warm showers, heating pads, warm or cool compresses, and self-massage of the affected area. Warm compresses can provide relief because moist heat has a penetrating effect that promotes healing and reduces soreness to a muscle area. Massage decreases muscle tension and can promote comfort. When providing comfort measures to patients in a psychiatric setting, the nurse should be mindful of using approaches that are appropriate for the patient's diagnosis, preferences, sense of dignity, and past trauma history. For example, comfort measures such as massage may not be appropriate for the patient experiencing paranoia or psychosis, or the patient with a history of sexual trauma. Less intimate types of comfort measures, such as cool compress, might be better tolerated. Based on the hospital's policies and procedures, some interventions require a doctor's order, as well as discussion and approval from the treatment team.

● Subgoal: Decrease the Patient's Pain-Related Anxiety

Assessment of the Patient's Pain-Related Anxiety
Unrelieved pain can increase anxiety; this anxiety can further compromise activities of daily living and can contribute to insomnia. Anxiety can also intensify the experience of pain, thus creating a vicious cycle. Research demonstrates that individuals with unusually high levels of anxiety also tend to have higher-than-normal perception of pain and a lower pain threshold (Leo, 2003; Massie, 2000). Moreover, individuals with an early experience of traumatic illness involving physical pain may be even more

anxious in the presence of pain, and they may experience pain more intensely (Leo, 2003; Massie, 2000).

In report. To understand the patient's fear and anxiety, the nurse should ask if there has been any change in level of agitation or other external signs of anxiety. The nurse can inquire about the patient's daily activities on the unit, sleep patterns, appetite, and interactions with others, as changes in these may suggest increased anxiety. If staff report that the patient has shown increased anxiety, the nurse may try to determine if there have been environmental or internal triggers to increase anxiety, distress, and fear. For example, the nurse may ask, "Has there been any change in pain or in the medical diagnosis or prognosis that could result in increased anxiety?"

One-to-one contact. During this contact, the nurse should take care to behave in a way that does not further increase anxiety. The nurse should use simple language that the patient can understand, and she should speak slowly and in a calm tone of voice. The nurse will sit facing the patient and at the same level if possible, so the nurse is in the patient's "field of vision." She can then ask more specific questions about anxiety, fear, and distress. The nurse should listen carefully to what the patient says. Is the patient expressing anxiety about her pain or other health-related anxiety? If so, the nurse may ask the patient, "What is the thing that scares you the most?" It is helpful to acknowledge that pain and anxiety frequently coexist and one experience can exacerbate the other. In doing so, the nurse also wants to be clear that both problems are "real" problems, and the relationship between pain and anxiety does not mean that the patient's pain is not real.

The nurse may also assess the extent to which patients have cognitions commonly associated with anxiety. For example, is the patient catastrophizing—does he say, "I will never be able to handle this pain" or "It will just get worse and worse and worse, and there is nothing I can do about it"?

On the unit. The nurse will observe the patient's behaviors on the unit. Does the patient exhibit nonverbal signs of anxiety, such as isolation, agitation, and refusal of food? Moreover, the nurse will determine whether the patient is attending and participating in group activities as anxiety may prevent this.

● Key Nursing Interventions to Decrease the Patient's Pain-Related Anxiety

Explore and challenge the patient's fears about pain. First, by listening and being present, the nurse can alleviate the patient's fear that her pain will not be taken seriously, thereby conveying a sense of legitimacy and self-worth to the patient. The nurse should always validate the pain or fear of pain first: "It makes sense that you are afraid you cannot handle your pain. You've had some very difficult months, so you are scared about the future." After acknowledging the patient's feelings, the nurse may then gently challenge the patient's fear. For example, the patient might be afraid to participate in a given activity because it could increase pain. The nurse can acknowledge that many individuals in pain are fearful of physical activity, and ask the patient "What is the worst thing about the pain that you are afraid of?" and "How bad would it be if that 'worst' thing happened?" The nurse can then suggest that sometimes the fear of experiencing the pain can be worse than the reality of the pain, and if able, the patient might consider trying the activity for a few minutes to test out that belief. (Note that the nurse will suggest that the patient take a small step in the direction of participating in a feared activity as this will seem less overwhelming to the patient.) Likewise, the nurse could ask about the pros and cons of remaining immobilized.

Teach or encourage the use of relaxation and distraction techniques. These techniques, discussed in Chapter 13, may not only help in alleviating pain, but may also help with associated anxiety.

Provide anxiety medications. The physician may choose to introduce an adjuvant medication, such as a benzodi-azepine. This may be appropriate in small doses to inhibit impulsive anxiety and allow the patient to participate more fully in other types of treatment.

● Subgoal: Help the Patient to Improve Functioning
   in the Presence of Pain

Assessment of Patient Functioning
Pain management is directed toward optimal pain relief, while at the same time promoting and improving functional capacity. "Good functioning" refers to performing tasks and activities that people find necessary or desirable in their lives, spanning from self-care and eating, to doing meaningful work and maintaining important relationships (Applegate, Blass, & Williams, 1990; Kane, R. L., & Kane, R. A., 2000). Maintaining or increasing functional capacity is critical to favorable outcomes and self esteem.

In report. The nurse will ascertain what the patient's functioning was prior to hospitalization. Is the patient's level of functioning better or worse than it was immediately before coming to the hospital? The nurse will also ask about the patient's level of functioning on the unit, including the patient's ability to perform activities for daily living (hygiene, dressing, eating, etc.), his participation in groups and unit activities, and whether the patient has articulated any feelings about his level of functioning. The nurse will listen for any significant change in the patient's functioning and organizational capabilities. Decreased functioning can affect the patient's safety, both affectively (e.g., increasing suicidal ideation) and physically (e.g., creating a higher risk for a fall).

One-to-one contact. When a patient's level of functioning has decreased significantly enough for her to be hospitalized for psychiatric reasons, it is important for the nurse to inquire about the patient's best level of functioning in the past, as well as expectations for the future. The nurse will ask specific questions about how the patient has been coping outside of the hospital. Was the patient able to take care of daily life activities, such as shopping for food, preparing meals, seeing friends and family, and working? How does the patient perceive her quality of life? What are the barriers to functioning? (The nurse may be surprised by the answer since pain may or may not be perceived by the patient to be a barrier to functioning.) The nurse will assess the individual's mobility, independence, and related factors such as sleep disturbances that may influence the person's ability to function. The nurse will also assess any avoidant behavior or unwillingness to participate in activities of daily living, such as eating, sleeping, dressing, and using the bathroom.

On the unit. The nurse will note the patient's functioning on the unit: is the patient eating, sleeping, and taking care of his own activities of daily living, including dressing, bathing, and grooming? Is he able to attend groups or participate in other unit programming?

● Key Nursing Interventions to Increase Functioning in the Presence of Pain

Assist patients with goal setting. As trust develops and the patient becomes more comfortable, the nurse may ask him about functional goals for the hospitalization and post hospital phase. To ensure that patient goals are realistic, individualized, and achievable, they should be developed collaboratively by both the patient and the team. An open-ended question for the patient is, "What two activities that you are not able to do now would you like to be able to do?" For one individual, dressing himself and walking to the bathroom may be a major step forward; another may want to be able to attend group meetings and participate in social activities on the inpatient unit. Even if pain persists, the nurse should encourage activity to the best of the patient's ability since the more the patient does, the better she will feel.

Reinforce functional activities; decrease focus on pain behaviors. The nurse can reinforce functional behavior through positive feedback. For example, the nurse may say, "I noticed you went to group today; I was glad to see that you were up to it" or "It looked like you enjoyed talking to X; I'm glad you started that conversation." The entire health care team should make efforts to focus on reinforcing functional behavior; this skill can also be taught to the family or those close to the patient.

Perhaps more challenging than reinforcing functional activities is avoiding the reinforcement of pain-related behaviors. Nurses listen intently to symptoms and naturally respond to overt behaviors. However, in some cases, being drawn into a monologue of symptom complaints and reacting to pain-related behaviors (i.e., behaviors such as continually rubbing a body part or groaning) can be counterproductive, serving only to reinforce the patient's focus on the pain. The patient then learns that talking about pain or behaving in a certain way brings attention to them. The nurse can manage this in a few ways. First, when the patient wants to talk about pain, the nurse can validate the patient's pain, determine whether any action is needed, and then move the conversation toward increasing functioning. It is very important not to skip the step of pain validation. For example, the nurse may say, "I'm sorry you are having such a hard time. I know your back really hurts.

I gave you your prn 15 minutes ago; let's wait a bit to see if it helps. In the meantime, I have been wanting to talk with you about your goals for your time on the unit. I notice you are going to group more often...." By refocusing the patient to the goals, the nurse has put great emphasis on the patient having some control over the plan and the outcome. Redirecting the patient toward goals may begin to allow the patient to recognize that taking an active role is expected and will produce better outcomes.

Second, regular assessments that are not driven by pain-related behaviors (rather, they occur at specified times) can help the nurse remain objective and help the patient feel cared for. At the same time, having regular assessments can break the association between the pain behaviors and the assessment (which may be reinforcing due to the attention from the nurse).

Third, the nurse may also try to help the patient understand that excessive talk about pain—to the exclusion of other topics—may discourage others from wanting to be close. The patient may not realize how his behavior is received or interpreted, or how it alienates others. If the patient can understand this, it may improve functioning of some of his relationships.

Support physical activity. Since the patient with pain may limit physical activity to avoid pain, the nurse may assist the patient in improving physical conditioning. The nurse will support the patient's involvement in an individualized program of exercise developed by the physical therapist or occupational therapist on the treatment team. This program of exercise should emphasize increased functioning, strength, flexibility, and endurance. The exercise program can be integrated with activities throughout the day on the unit. The nurse will encourage the patient to be out of bed during the day, providing positive reinforcement for involvement in unit activities. The nurse will monitor physiologic responses to increased activity level, including respiration, heart rate and rhythm, and blood pressure. He may encourage the patient to walk on the unit, perhaps down one hallway, or half a hallway to start, gradually increasing the distance each day. While encouraging more activity, the nurse should also identify and minimize factors that cause fatigue. Most patients do not understand that inactivity can actually increase pain and that movement and exercise, however minimal it may be, are important aspects of pain treatment.

As part of the exercise program, the nurse may adopt a cognitive approach by asking about the person's fears and beliefs about the movement or activity they are undertaking. Frequently, this will demonstrate that the person's caution relates to fear of further damage. This fear may not be realistic, and the nurse can offer appropriate information that may help combat this fear. It is also critical that the nurse remind the patient that although physical activity may increase pain in the short term, it may actually serve to decrease pain in the long term.

Teach sleep hygiene. Sleep disturbance is common among individuals with pain, and lack of sleep can interfere with daily functioning. Therefore, the nurse may educate the patient to take rest periods to facilitate comfort, sleep, relaxation, recovery, and work and family functioning. The nurse can also (1) teach the patient to use relaxation exercises at bedtime and if awakened during the night, (2) suggest the patient take a warm shower or develop other personal hygiene routines prior to bedtime, (3) suggest the patient read a book before bed to distract from negative thoughts, and (4) recommend the patient to avoid or minimize caffeine, omitting it entirely after 6 p.m. In the evening, the nurse can provide milk and a high-protein snack, such as cheese, to promote sleep. Finally, nursing staff will want to create a quiet, restful environment by keeping the unit milieu calm and quiet during evening and bedtime hours.

TREATMENT ENGAGEMENT

● **Subgoal: Engage the Patient in Treatment Despite the Experience of Pain**

Assessment of Patient Engagement in Treatment

As depression, fear, and anxiety experienced decreases and the pain itself is reduced, the patient's ability to engage in treatment should improve. To assess the degree of engagement on the unit, the nurse will consider the following questions: "Is the patient participating in activities of daily living with more independence and less encouragement?" "How much time does the patient spend out of her room?" "Is she willingly socializing with others on the unit?" "Is she out in the milieu more frequently, eating meals with others, and attending any groups?" "Is she taking her medications regularly?" The nurse will look for other outcomes to assess whether the patient has engaged in treatment, for example, whether the patient has an increased understanding of the way pain, anxiety, and depression interconnect, and whether the patient is able to apply or request help with adaptive coping strategies for pain and associated anxiety or distress.

If patient's engagement in treatment is not proceeding as expected or desired, the nurse should assess the barriers. Two common barriers to engagement are (1) experiencing frustration and mistrust of health care providers due to a history of medical disappointments for pain relief, and (2) using "physical pain talk" as a way to avoid examination of problems in life or psychiatric symptoms.

● **Key Nursing Interventions to Increase Engagement in Treatment**

Respect and listen to the patient; accept her physical pain as real. The patient in pain often feels disrespected and disempowered. Previous health care providers or family members may have told the patient that her pain is not real and it is all "in her head," or that she is just exaggerating. Therefore, during all contacts, it is very important that the nurse use a nonjudgmental, matter-of-fact, courteous, and interested approach to foster trust and encourage engagement. The nurse should express willingness to help and consistently communicate that even if the cause of the pain is unknown or poorly understood, he understands that the pain is very real. The nurse's focus should be on the patient's subjective experience of pain and the impact the pain has on the patient's life. She may tell the patient, "I know your pain is real, and I'm sorry that you have to experience so much pain." As mentioned earlier, providing prn pain medication as ordered and using other pain-relief strategies assures the patient that the nurse accepts that the pain is real.

If the patient has been frustrated by past providers and expresses mistrust in caregivers, the nurse should allow him to talk about these feelings, and to have time to tell the nurse the "story" of what they have been through in the quest to obtain relief. The nurse will listen to the patient's frustrations in a nonjudgmental manner, while taking care not to criticize or undermine any other providers. Rather, the nurse will listen to the patient's past treatment experiences and empathize only with their long, arduous journey (e.g., "It sounds like you have been through a lot in the past and have been in pain for a long time"). From this encounter, the nurse can begin to shift the focus to what has been helpful and less helpful with previous treatment attempts, emphasizing that each provider must learn from and build upon past experience. Then, the nurse can emphasize that this hospitalization is a new experience with new opportunities. To foster ownership and responsibility, the nurse will invite the patient to actively participate in crafting the care plan, and openly communicate as modifications need to be made. Finally, the nurse needs to acknowledge that this journey is profoundly challenging, both physically and emotionally. Embarking on this journey and remaining on course, despite the inevitable obstacles, indeed takes enormous courage.

Help the patient recognize and accept the relationship between his pain and psychiatric symptoms. Excessive "physical pain talk" can be a major obstacle to engagement in treatment, improvements in functioning, or talking about emotions. That is, the patient may talk about pain exclusively, and refuse to focus on other life issues. If a patient is not psychotic, is cognitively intact, and exhibits insight, the nurse can try to address his focus on the pain to the exclusion of talking about feelings or fears. The nurse may say, "I know you are feeling a great deal of pain in your back, and it must be really tough to be going through that. But I wonder it seems like it might also be important to talk about the loss you've recently experienced." In contrast, with more fragile populations such as cognitively impaired patients—patients with active psychotic or paranoid symptoms or on suicide watch—the nurse should be cautious in addressing deeper emotional issues, as this may cause agitation, loss of trust, or self-harming behaviors.

When the nurse is unsure how to help the patient refocus on life problems and feelings rather than solely on physical pain, it is always best to communicate with the treatment team and work together to choose the best approach to help the patient gain insight.

PREPARATION FOR DISCHARGE

Discuss medication use. It is of utmost importance that the patient understands the postdischarge medication regimen. The nurse should provide clear instructions about medication administration not only for pain medication but also for all medications prescribed. Ideally, the nurse, along with key treatment team members, should meet with the patient (and significant supports) before discharge. This type of meeting is routine in most inpatient psychiatric hospital settings. At this meeting, a written list of medications should be provided, including dosage, frequency, description of what each medication is for, and importance of keeping the medications in a safe location away from children, pets, and family members or friends with potential suicidal tendencies. The nurse should explain what the patient could do if uncomfortable side effects are experienced or if any medication questions arise after discharge. Clear instructions for follow-up visits are crucial, whether it is with the patient's primary care physician or a pain management referral. These patients need guidance and encouragement on an ongoing basis for continued success. Outpatient psychiatric and physical therapy programs may also provide better follow through and treatment outcomes.

Discuss options for pain relief with the patient for the posthospitalization period. The nurse may also explore the patient's willingness or ability to explore a broad range of techniques aimed at controlling pain post discharge. Medications and relaxation have been discussed previously. The nurse may discuss cognitive behavioral therapy (CBT) with the patient. CBT has demonstrated efficacy in treating patients with pain (Turk, Meichenbaum, & Genest, 1983; Wells-Federman, Arnstein, & Caudill, 2002). CBT includes cognitive restructuring in which patients learn to identify and challenge negative thinking patterns and develop more adaptive, coping thoughts. CBT also includes teaching behavioral techniques such as progressive relaxation and other brief relaxation exercises to decrease muscle tension, reduce emotional distress, and divert attention from pain; time-based pacing to ensure that patients do not "overdo it," resulting in periods of increased pain; problem-solving; sleep hygiene; goal setting; and communication training (Keefe & Gil, 1986).

In addition, the nurse may also explore the patient's interest and experience with integrative medicine approaches (also called "adjunctive medicine") that are intended to bring forth relaxation and healing and reduce pain. Some examples of adjunctive treatments that have demonstrated efficacy for some pain conditions are reiki, acupuncture, and massage. Reiki is a Japanese technique for stress reduction and relaxation. Research shows that reiki can reduce anxiety, muscle tension, and pain, as well as promote accelerated wound healing and wellness and a greater sense of well-being (Berman, 2004; Richeson, Spross, Lutz, & Peng, 2010). Acupuncture, which is based on ancient Chinese medicine, involves the process of inserting very fine needles to the various acupuncture points on the body. Acupuncture promotes physical and emotional well-being, and with this, a reduction in pain (American Pain Foundation, 2010; Berman, 2004). Finally, therapeutic massage can increase blood circulation to the muscles, decrease stress, decrease muscle tension, and improve range of motion (Ernst, 2004). As an example, one randomized, controlled trial examined the impact of massage with 605 adult patients undergoing abdominal or thoracic surgery. Results showed that patients receiving massage therapy every day in the postoperative hospital stay had overall improvements in pain relief and anxiety (Mitchinson et al., 2007).

We do note that although there is some evidence that some of these alternative approaches relieve pain and increase the pain threshold, it is recommended they be used in conjunction with traditional pain-relief methods. The nurse will always advise the patient to let her provider know about adjunctive therapies being used.

TABLE 6.1
Goals, Areas of Assessment, and Interventions for a Patient With Pain

Goal	Assessment	Intervention
Safety		
Prevent or reduce the risk for harm to self	Know that the presence of chronic pain increases risk for suicide ideation and behavior Identify and communicate suicide risk factors in report and team meetings Assess patient's suicide risk using direct inquiry Monitor medication to ensure it is not being "cheeked"	Create a safe environment for the patient Discourage isolation Express realistic hope about the future Treat the physical pain
Stabilization		
Reduce or alleviate pain symptoms	Assess pain intensity and severity regularly via self-report if possible; otherwise via observation Use a rating scale to track and document pain severity over time Monitor vital signs and related physical symptoms Watch for isolative behaviors on the unit	Assist physician with finding the source of pain and selecting effective interventions Administer medication to reduce or alleviate pain Teach about medications Teach the patient to accurately report her pain Teach relaxation and distraction techniques Provide nursing comfort measures
Decrease the patient's pain-related anxiety	Assess level of anxiety related to pain using direct inquiry and observation Assess pain-related catastrophizing	Explore and challenge patient's fears about pain Teach or encourage use of relaxation or distraction techniques Provide anxiety medications

(cont.)

TABLE 6.1
Goals, Areas of Assessment, and Interventions for a
Patient With Pain   *(cont.)*

Goal	Assessment	Intervention
Stabilization		
Help patient to improve functioning in the presence of pain	Assess level of functioning, including ability to complete activities of daily life, and home and work responsibilities, prior to hospitalization Observe level of functioning in the hospital	Assist patients with goal setting Reinforce functional activities; decrease focus on pain behaviors Support physical activity Teach sleep hygiene
Treatment Engagement		
Engage the patient in treatment despite the experience of pain	Assess patient's degree of engagement in unit activities and treatment Look for barriers to engagement, including mistrust of health care providers, and using "physical pain talk" as a way to avoid talking about other difficult topics	Respect and listen to patient; accept her physical pain as real Help patient recognize and accept relationship between his pain and psychiatric symptoms

REFERENCES

Adams, N., Poole, H., & Richardson, C. (2006). Psychological approach to chronic pain management: Part I. *Issues in Clinical Nursing, 15*, 290–300.

American Pain Foundation. (2010). Topic brief: Integrative medicine: non-drug treatment options for pain management. Retrieved October 12, 2010, from http://www.painfoundation.org/search/integrativemedicine

American Psychiatric Association. (2000). *Diagnostic and statistical manual of mental disorders: DSM IV-TR*. Washington, DC: Author.

Applegate, W. B., Blass, J. P., & Williams, T. E. (1990). Instruments for the functional assessment of older patients. *New England Journal of Medicine, 322*(17), 1132–1148.

Berman, B. (2004). Is it just a case of more tools for the medical bag? *Clinical Journal of Pain 20* (1), 1–2

Dewar, A., Osborne, M., Mullett, J., Langdeau, S., & Plummer, M. (2009). Psychiatric patients: How can we decide if you are in pain? *Issues in Mental Health Nursing, 30*, 295–303.

Ernst, E. (2004). Manual therapies for pain control: Chiropractic and massage. *Clinical Journal of Pain, 20*(1), 8–12.

Gatchel, R. (2004a). *Clinical essentials of pain management.* Washington, DC: American Psychological Association.

Gatchel, R. (2004b). Comorbidity of chronic pain and mental health disorders: The biopsychosocial perspective. *American Psychologist, 59*(8), 795–805.

Gatchel, R., & Turk, D. (1999). *Psychosocial factors in pain: Critical perspectives.* New York: The Guilford Press.

Horgas, A., Nichols, A., Schapson, C., &Vietes, K. (2007). Assessing pain in persons with dementia: Relationships among the noncommunicative patient's pain assessment instrument, self-report, and behavioral observations. *Pain Management Nursing, 8*(2), 77–85.

International Association of the Study of Pain. (2010). Retrieved November 15, 2010, from http://www.iasp-pain.org

Kane, R. L., & Kane, R. A. (2000). *Assessing older persons: Measurement, meaning, and practical applications.* New York: Oxford University Press.

Keefe, F. J., & Gil, K. M. (1986). Behavioral concepts in the analysis of chronic pain syndromes. *Journal of Consulting and Clinical Psychology, 54*, 776–783.

Lancee, W., Vachon, M., Ghadirian, P., Adair, W., Conway, B., & Dryer, D. (1994). The impact of pain and impaired role performance on distress in persons with cancer. *Canadian Journal of Psychiatry, 39*, 617–622.

Lasch, K.E. (2000). Culture, pain, and culturally sensitive pain care. *Pain Management Nursing, 1*(3) Suppl 1, 16–22.

Leo, R. (2003). *Pain management for psychiatrists.* Washington, DC: American Psychiatric Publishing.

Massie, M. (2000). *Pain: What psychiatrists need to know.* Washington, DC: American Psychiatric Press, Inc.

Massie, M., & Holland, J. (1990). Depression and the cancer patient. *Journal of Clinical Psychiatry, 51*, 12–17.

Melzack, R, & Wall. P. D. (1965). Pain mechanisms: A new theory. *Science, 150* (699), 971–979

Mitchinson, A. R., Kim, H. M., Rosenberg, J, M., Geisser, M., Kirsh, M., Cikrit, D., & Hinshaw, D. B. (2007). Acute postoperative pain management using massage as an adjuvant therapy. *Archives of Surgery, 142*(12), 1158–1167.

Narayan, M. (2010). Culture's effects on pain assessment and management. *American Journal of Nursing, 110*(4), 38–47.

Payen, J. (2001). Pain is assessed in the critically ill sedated patients using a behavioral pain scale. *Critical Care Medicine, 29*(12), 2258–2263.

Richeson, N.E., Spross, J.A., Lutz, K., & Peng, C. (2010). Effects of Reiki on anxiety, depression, pain, and physiological factors in community-dwelling older adults. *Research in Gerontological Nursing, 3*(3), 187–99.

Simon, J. M. (1996). Chronic pain syndrome: Nursing assessment and intervention. *Rehabilitation Nursing, 21*(1), 13–19.

St. Marie, B. (Ed.). (2002). *American society of pain management nurses: Core curriculum for pain management nursing.* Philadelphia, PA: W.B. Saunders Publishing Co.

Tang, N., & Crane, C. (2006). Suicidality in chronic pain: A review of the prevalence, risk factors and psychological links. *Psychological Medicine, 36*, 575–586.

Townsend, M. (2006). *Psychiatric mental health nursing: Concepts of care in evidence-based practice* (5th ed.). Philadelphia, PA: F.A. Davis Company.

Turk, D. C., Meichenbaum, D., & Genest, M. (1983). Pain and behavioral medicine: A cognitive-behavioral perspective. New York: Guilford Press.

Webster, L., & Dove, B. (2007). Avoiding opioid abuse while managing pain. North Branch, MI: Sunrise River Press.

Wells- Federman, C., Arnstein, P. & Caudill, M. (2002). Nurse-led pain management program: Effect on self-efficacy, pain intensity, pain-related disability, and depressive symptoms in chronic pain patients. *Pain Management Nursing, 3*(4), 131–140.

The Patient With Paranoia   7

Joanne M. Matthew, Judy L. Sheehan,
Lisa A. Uebelacker, Laura Drury,
Linda Damon, and Patricia R. Recupero

BACKGROUND AND DESCRIPTION

Behavior

The patient exhibiting paranoid behaviors may present as socially withdrawn and unwilling to engage in conversation, or, alternatively, as aggressive (Herzog & Varcarolis, 2010). Sometimes, one patient may fluctuate between the two extremes. They may have trouble interacting with groups of people, often getting into disagreements with others that may quickly escalate into aggression. On the other hand, the patient may avoid interaction with others while at the same time pacing the unit and vigilantly scanning the environment. There are patients who will sit or sleep in carefully selected and specific locations in public areas and become upset if the space is not available to them. The patient with paranoid behaviors may not eat meals with the community and prefer to isolate. This patient may refuse food, fluids, and medications even if this creates a potential health problem. These behaviors, which are driven by beliefs that he is in danger of being harmed in some way, are often frightening and concerning to the community at large.

Cognition

The behavior described above often has an underlying logic once one understands the cognitions behind it. The patient with paranoia often has a strong distrust of others and thinks she may be harmed. Her delusional thinking may include beliefs that she is being watched, followed, poisoned, or persecuted (Williams, 1990). These thoughts may be expressed in language as "I know you are trying to kill me," "That medication is poison," "This isn't really a hospital, you are all actors," "Everyone is talking about me," or "I know there is a camera in my room." This individual may interpret environmental stimuli as proof of this delusional thinking. For example, a patient may consider a change in the color of her medication to be evidence to support a persecutory belief (Williams, 1990).

Affect

The patient with paranoia may look and feel afraid or angry. It is important to understand how frightened and anxious this patient may feel even if it is not evident in his external expression (Herzog & Varacolis, 2010). The intensity of the underlying affect and the associated cognitions can make any situation, no matter how seemingly simple and benign, potentially complicated and explosive.

Context

Paranoid behavior in psychiatric inpatients is often a symptom of a potentially treatable psychotic process as opposed to a particular personality or relational style. Paranoia is a common symptom of many psychiatric and/or medical diagnoses, including schizophrenia, bipolar disorder (manic, mixed, or depressed episodes), major depression with psychotic features, substance-induced psychotic disorder, delusional disorder, posttraumatic stress disorder, psychotic disorder due to medical condition, and organic brain disease (APA, 2005). Although this list is not all-inclusive, the wide variety of conditions explains why nurses frequently observe paranoid behaviors on the inpatient unit.

POTENTIAL BARRIERS TO BEING THERAPEUTIC

The patient with paranoid behaviors can be difficult to approach, may respond angrily to interventions, and will not automatically trust the nurse to be helpful. Interacting with these individuals can generate feelings of fear, frustration, helplessness, or anger for the nurse. Intervening successfully with this patient requires the nurse to control her own affective response so that her emotions do not fuel the patient's fear (Herzog & Varcarolis, 2010). Nurses must be patient, as interventions can take longer with these individuals. The nurse may feel pressure to get tasks completed, but translating that urgency to the patient by speaking rapidly or appearing rushed can defeat efforts to build trust with this patient. The patient may perceive that pressure as coercive and as evidence for a belief that there is a "hidden agenda" underlying a given intervention that is not beneficial to the patient.

Consequently, the nurse needs to identify when his own anxiety or frustration may be transmitted to the patient, and whenever possible, he should attempt to remain outwardly calm, and take a break if necessary. The nurse can remind himself that he is dealing with a very frightened individual. It can be helpful to remember that this person is suffering from a serious disease that affects all of their perceptions.

The dynamic nature of the inpatient environment challenges the nurse to think quickly, act deliberately, and usually target more than one goal at a time. This is important because as anxiety is reduced, the risk of harm to self or others is also reduced and engagement in treatment becomes more likely (Williams, 1990). Thus, even though managing dangerousness is a priority, many of the primary nursing interventions will focus on reducing the patient's levels of anxiety, often through interventions that allow him to develop an increasing level of trust in the nurse and in his other health care providers, thus increasing engagement in treatment (Herzog & Varcarolis, 2010).

One of the particular challenges of working with paranoid patients is that there might be a conflict between the needs of the individual (for reaching therapeutic goals) and the needs the community. The nurse must choose the timing and type of interventions in order to provide for the safety of all the patients on the unit. For example, intervening too soon to prevent a potential aggressive act may cause the patient to feel controlled or precipitate further aggression. Intervening too late may create more feelings of fear and lack of safety for the other patients on the unit. The nurse, who must manage these potentially divergent needs, must continually reevaluate the situation and be flexible in approach (Delaney & Johnson, 2006; Johnson & Delaney, 2007).

OVERVIEW OF NURSING CARE GOALS

1. Safety
   - Prevent aggression toward others
   - Prevent active self-harm
   - Prevent passive self-harm
2. Stabilization
   - Decrease fear and anxiety
3. Engagement
   - Increase engagement in treatment

SAFETY

● Subgoal: Prevent Aggression Toward Others

Patients experiencing paranoia are at increased risk for aggression (Schultz, North, & Shields, 2007). That being said, although many paranoid patients exhibit some of the warning signs described below, such as agitation, many never harm themselves or others.

Assessment of Risk for Aggression Toward Others

In report. Proactive assessment of risk begins prior to meeting the patient. On hearing that a patient is "paranoid" or has "paranoid symptoms," the nurse will consider the following: What is the person's history? History of aggression is one factor that is known to increase the probability that a person is at risk to harm others. Is there a history of an isolated incident or have there been several episodes? A greater number of past occurrences will increase the risk of aggression occurring again. Has the patient been destructive to property? Is the patient experiencing command hallucinations? These factors also increase the risk for aggressive behavior. What is the patient's diagnosis? Patients who are schizophrenic or have impulse control problems are at greater risk for aggressive behaviors. Does the patient have an organic brain disease or a neurologic impairment? These individuals are also at greater risk for aggression (Quanbeck & McDermott, 2008).

One-to-one contact. The patient's response to the very first interactions with the nurse will provide an initial measure of the patient's ability to tolerate other people. Those with a low tolerance for interactions may be at higher risk for aggression toward others (Murphy & Carson, 2010). The nurse will need to gauge the appropriate distance to maintain, the best location of the initial interview, and the need for staff assistance. The nurse may allow the patient to choose the location and placement of the seating for the interview. In addition to making the patient more comfortable, this can provide important information how the patient perceives others in her environment. During the interview, the nurse will consider questions related to comfort with interpersonal interactions, such as "Can the person participate in the entire interview?" "How easily does the individual engage in conversation?" "How much space does the patient put between himself and the person conducting the interview?"

During this interview, the nurse will be looking for non-verbal indicators of agitation, as agitation may indicate an increased risk for aggression toward others. Agitation or anxiety may be expressed as vigilant scanning of the environment, pacing, appearing restless, or having a clenched jaw, rigid posture, or fixed, tense facial expression. Physiological indicators such as rapid breathing and sweating may also indicate an increasingly agitated state (Murphy & Carson, 2010).

The initial conversation with a patient demonstrating paranoid behavior may be brief and appear somewhat casual. The nurse should keep questions to a minimum if possible, and questions should be clear and offered to the patient one at a time. The nurse will start with a general question such as "How are you doing?" or "How do you feel about being here?" The nurse should also directly ask the person if she hears voices. For example, "Are you hearing voices other than mine or the people around us?" "What do they say to you?" If the patient does not respond, the nurse can ask, "Do you hear voices telling you not to talk with me?" If auditory hallucinations are indeed present, then it is important to ask what the voices say. For example, the nurse may ask, "What are they saying to you?" "Are they telling you to hurt yourself or someone else?" If the patient denies voices or refuses to answer but begins to fidget or become increasingly anxious, this *may* indicate that voices are indeed present. Whereas command hallucinations are not a direct cause of patient aggression, there is some evidence that the patient's emotional response to the hallucinations may increase the risk that he would act upon the commands (Braham et al., 2004). The nurse should also keep in mind that, as important as it is to become familiar with the patient's internal experience, pushing for answers with a paranoid patient may hinder the development of a thera- peutic relationship and stimulate an aggressive response. Some very paranoid patients may not be able to engage in a conversation.

On the unit. The nurse will attempt to assess and under- stand how the patient is interpreting even the most benign or routine activities on the unit. Obviously, a patient who is shouting to other people to leave her "stuff" alone, or saying "don't talk about me" or "you better not come near me" is demonstrating defensive behavior, which could precede aggressive acts. The nurse may also notice more subtle indicators of agitation such as glaring or darting eye contact or even visual scanning. Visual scanning, or the eyes moving rapidly from side to side in a monitor- ing motion, may occur in the context of the patient's body remaining rigid and may indicate an increasing level of agitation.

This patient may spend time on the unit (as opposed to her room) because she feels the need to monitor the environment. Therefore, the nurse may observe that this patient will sit in a chair that is against a wall in order to be able to view everyone that approaches. Alternatively, she may want to stay in her room. As an example, a patient may arrange her bedroom with her bed up against a wall, and sit in her room, on her bed with her back to the wall in order to watch everyone who comes in and out of the room.

● Key Nursing Interventions to Prevent Aggression Toward Others

If the nurse assesses the patient as becoming a risk to the safety of others, there are several interventions she may use. In choosing from among the interventions, the nurse will consider (1) the patient's ability to communicate what he or she is afraid of and what he or she believes will help decrease risk of aggression; (2) what has worked with this patient in the past; and (3) how imminent is the risk of aggression. Once the nurse has developed a relationship with the patient, the patient may be able to tell the nurse, "I feel like hurting someone" or "I need to get away from ...." Then, the nurse may have the opportunity to elicit the patient's preferences for distracting or calming activities and collaborate with the patient on a strategy to manage the patient's distress.

Offer verbal reassurance. If the patient is yelling at staff or other patients while out on the unit, the nurse can respond initially to the fear the patient may be expressing. For example, if a patient is yelling "get away from me...stop following me," the nurse can begin his interventions by reassuring the patient that she is safe and no one is going to hurt her. This simple intervention can sometimes defuse a potentially volatile situation.

Modify the environment and reduce demands. Sometimes the nurse will determine that the patient is most at risk for harming others during specific situations such as meals or group activities, or in response to specific triggers. Potentially volatile situations can be avoided if the nurse caring for the individual modifies the environment whenever possible and places fewer demands on the patient. For example, the nurse may bring food or medications to the patient instead of having the patient in the larger milieu. The nurse may choose not to insist that the patient comes out of his room, joins in group activities, or engages in lengthy one-to-one contact. If the patient has chosen a particular area of the unit to sit, nursing staff can respect that choice and try to keep that area open for the patient. Asking other people, such as visitors and other patients, to allow the person some space and privacy may minimize the risk to others.

Provide sensory interventions. Sensory interventions can help to calm or distract a paranoid patient, thereby reducing her risk of harm to others. See Chapter 14 for suggested sensory interventions, including the open door quiet room.

Provide space and privacy. In order to reduce a patient's agitation, as well as to increase a sense of safety among other patients, the nurse may want to direct a patient who is demonstrating high levels of psychomotor agitation to a quieter space. The nurse must approach this patient cautiously. Some quiet areas to choose on the inpatient unit include the patient's room, the sensory room, the open-door quiet room, or a quieter end of the unit. The nurse can say to the patient, "Please come with me to...," or "You seem to be having a hard time, let's go someplace quieter." The nurse may give the patient a choice of where to go that is quieter. However, if the nurse determines that the patient is an imminent risk of harm to others, then the nurse will have to give the patient more direct instruction. For the highest risk patient, or the patient who does not respond to an initial request and continues to behave in a frightening way, the nurse will want to enlist other staff to approach the patient with him. Staff could then directly tell the patient that they want her to take some time in a quieter space. Although there is always a risk that having several staff approach the patient at once will make the patient more agitated, the nurse must also maintain his own safety and show that the staff is uniformly concerned about the patient's behavior. The patient may experience this as intimidating, but it is preferable to physical restraint.

Offer prn medication. The prn medication can be used to treat the agitation or psychotic symptoms that may contribute to risk for aggression. Before discussing this intervention option, we want to acknowledge that this can be a controversial topic and that different hospitals and physicians have different standards regarding prn medications. Therefore, the suggestions presented here may need to be modified in order to be appropriate for a particular setting. It is always appropriate, however, to request that a physician clarify when and how prn medications should be used.

The prn medications that may be appropriate include antipsychotic medications and benzodiazepines (Krawkowski et al., 2006; Quanbeck, 2006). When deciding on whether to offer the patient the prn medication and which medication to offer, the nurse will follow the physician's orders and consider the physician's rationale, as well as consider what worked well for the patient in the past, the current level of agitation, and whether the patient's behavior is in response to hallucinations or delusions. If the patient is very agitated and is having trouble processing stimulation from the external environment, or is actively hallucinating, he may benefit from a prn antipsychotic. These medications may also be useful when a patient has not been taking his prescribed antipsychotic medications prior to the current admission and/or is known to have had an idiosyncratic reaction to a benzodiazepine, such as increased aggressiveness or disinhibition (Quanbeck, 2006). If the patient is further along in his stay and has been taking his regularly scheduled antipsychotic medication for at least a few days, the nurse may want to try the benzodiazepine; this may help the patient's fear and anxiety. Offering both types of medications at once may be beneficial if the nurse assesses that the patient is at a greater level of risk to others (i.e., is extremely agitated). Initially, the nurse will offer oral (po) medications. However, if the nurse determines that the risk of harm to others is imminent and the patient is refusing the oral medication, then administering the medication parenterally by intramuscular injection may be required. See Chapter 12 for ways to approach the patient with medications.

Use containment as a last resort. Restraint and/or seclusion are rarely seen as therapeutic by the patient who experiences it. It is not strictly a nursing intervention as it requires physician consultation and a physician's order. However, nurses are the one type of professional who must contribute to a decision regarding the use of restraint or seclusion in the inpatient setting. Restraint or seclusion is used only in situations where the interventions already discussed do not work, or when the potential for aggression escalates very quickly due to the severity of the patient's condition. Hospital policy and procedure for restraint and seclusion determines the nurse's actions. Note that before, during, and after this intervention, the nurse will continue to try to engage the patient in the hope that as the severity of the patient's symptoms lessens, the patient will be able to work with the nurse in developing less restrictive methods to manage her aggressive urges. Please see also Chapter 16, "Managing Violence."

● Subgoal: Prevent Active Self-Harm

Active self-harm can include both injury with intent to kill oneself and self-injurious behaviors without intent to kill oneself. We cover the topic of working with the suicidal patient in Chapter 9. Here we focus primarily on self-harm without suicidal intent although some of the discussion will certainly apply to any type of self-harm. Although there is also a chapter (Chapter 5) on nonsuicidal self-injury, the type of NSSI that the paranoid patient engages in is often in response to psychotic delusions or hallucinations, in particular ones with religious or sexual themes, and can be memorable and often extreme. There are examples of these patients attempting self-castration, self-enucleation, or burning themselves with hot liquids or cigarettes (Favazza & Rosenthal, 1993). However, nonsuicidal self-harm is also very rare in this patient population (Favazza & Rosenthal, 1993), and for that reason, can be difficult to predict.

Assessment of Risk for Active Self-Harm
In report. The nurse's assessment of the potential for self-harm begins when he or she hears the report. When trying to determine whether the person may actively attempt to harm him- or herself, previous history may be an important indicator. Therefore, the nurse will want to know whether the patient has recently engaged in any self-destructive behavior, and if so, what were the circumstances, means, and outcome. In addition, the nurse will want to know what kinds of delusions the patient may be experiencing (Favazza & Rosenthal, 1990).

One-to-one contact. During the one-to-one contact, the nurse will want to assess for agitation, as this may be associated with self-harm, and ask direct questions about psychotic processes that may contain content related to self-harm. In particular, the nurse will want to ask if the patient is experiencing command hallucinations and ask about the content of their delusions. Please see Chapter 15, "Therapeutic One to One," for more information about assessing agitation and psychotic content one to one with these patients.

On the unit. The nurse will want to assess a patient who has paranoid thoughts and is at risk for self-harm at frequent intervals. Again, it is difficult to know what may indicate an increased risk for self-harm, but possible behaviors to look for are increased agitation, crying or visible anger, or isolation or lack of communication (Yearwood & Shoemaker, 2010).

● Key Nursing Interventions to Prevent Active Self-Harm

Administer medications. Agitation and psychotic symptoms may contribute to risk for self-harm; therefore, prn medications can be useful in this instance. (Please see Chapter 12 for information on how and when to choose a prn medication.)

Increase monitoring. The nurse will determine if the patient requires increased observation. In consultation with the patient's physician and/or the nurse's direct supervisor, the nurse can decide what level is required, such as suicide precautions or constant observation. It can be difficult to assess what level of observation will be helpful because a paranoid individual will feel threatened by someone following her around as is required in one-to-one observation. The patient may not understand why the bathroom has to be locked, as in special precautions. A decrease in privacy may, in fact, increase agitation or reinforce the patient's belief that she is being watched or followed, as psychotic symptoms may impair the paranoid patient's ability to rationally comprehend staff's reasons for following her or restricting her movements. Further, a single staff member doing the closer supervision may not be physically able to prevent the individual from harming herself. The most that the staff member may be able to do is alert other staff. That being said, the benefit of closer monitoring is that it can decrease the opportunities for the patient to harm herself and it allows staff to exert more control over the environment.

When increased monitoring does need to occur, it is important that staff communicate clearly and respectfully. The nurse should include the patient in discussions about keeping him safe from self-harm in order to provide the patient the opportunity to interpret the monitoring as concern for his safety. The nurse should greet the patient by name each time she observes the patient, ask the patient if he needs anything, and repeatedly make it clear that the intention is to be helpful.

Modify the environment. If the patient has a specific intent or action plan, in spite of a closer observation, the nurse can try to remove items from the unit environment or further restrict the patient's access to certain areas. For example, if the patient is using hot water to harm herself, then staff can remove the teakettle or lock the kitchen area. Interventions such as these can be drastic and involve limiting all of the patients' access to specific areas and items; therefore, the nurse's consultation with supervisors and physician is essential.

Use containment as a last resort. In the event that the other interventions fail, the nurse must consider whether restraint or seclusion is urgently needed to keep the patient safe. Please see Chapter 5, "The Patient With Nonsuicidal Self-Injury," for more information on the use of this intervention.

● Subgoal: Prevent Passive Self-Harm

Although active nonsuicidal self-injury in a patient with paranoia is less frequent, the risk for passive self-harm for this individual is more common (Williams, 1990). A person with paranoid beliefs or thoughts may be afraid to eat, drink, or care for primary hygienic needs. Patients with preexisting medical conditions may be unable to maintain required self-care routines. For example, a patient with diabetes may not adhere to dietary restrictions or take their medications because he does not believe that he is diabetic. The patient who has hypertension may think that health care providers have lied about his diagnosis, and therefore believe that he is not hypertensive and does not need treatment. Some patients may be afraid of the shower or water based on beliefs about poisonous gases or cameras in the shower.

Assessment of Risk for Passive Self-Harm
In report. Key questions to ask in report include, "Has this person been eating or drinking?" "Has she lost weight

recently?" "Are there any hygiene issues?" "When has she last showered or changed her clothing?" "Has any of the staff noticed any odors, lice, or stains?" "Has the patient been taking medications for her medical conditions?" These questions will help determine the degree of bio-physical risk for the patient.

One-to-one contact. During the one-to-one contact, the nurse should be aware of any odors, stains on the cloth-ing, matted hair, dirty hands and fingernails, and poten-tially open wounds, as these provide critical information about the patient's health and well-being. The nurse may ask, "I have noticed you have not been eating. Can you tell me about that?" or "I wonder if there is some reason you have not taken a shower recently." Although the patient's response may not be accurate or based on reality, it may provide some insight or information to the nurse.

On the unit. Monitoring the person's vital signs, intake, output, and weight will provide a measure of his physical status before a crisis occurs. However, a paranoid patient may not allow this type of monitoring. If this is the case, it will be important to observe the amount of food and fluid taken at meals, noting any empty food cartons in the trash or observing for meals taken with visitors as ways to assess intake.

● **Key Nursing Interventions to Prevent Passive Self-Harm**

The main objectives are ensuring that the patient is taking necessary medications, food, and fluids, as well as attend-ing to at least minimal hygiene needs.

Meet nutritional needs. First, the nurse will want to *provide a clear rationale and offer reassurance.* For example, if the patient was recently hospitalized for dehydration, the nurse may say, "You need to drink to stay healthy;

we do not want you to have to go back to the hospital." A clear rationale may not be effective if the patient is acting on delusional beliefs, but it is important to attempt it. The rationale may make more sense to the patient as delusional/paranoid beliefs subside. Sometimes, it can be helpful to express concern for the patient. For example, the nurse may say, "We are really worried about you because you haven't had anything to eat for a few days."

The second key type of intervention is *offering choices.* For example, the nurse might say, "I can see that you are having a hard time trusting us. Would it help if I opened this in front of you or let you open it yourself?" Patients will often accept food if it is individually wrapped, if it is opened in front of them, or if it is a preferred food. The nurse will want to be sure that the patient can choose a type of food that he feels comfortable eating. If the patient cannot verbalize this himself, family members can provide information about food preferences, so the staff can make these particular choices available to the patient. It can be helpful if the hospital provides food in sealed containers (Herzog & Varcarolis, 2010). This can be reassuring to the individual who fears malicious tampering of the food. Along these same lines, hospitals often have individual containers of cereal or crackers, juice, or milk; the patient may fell more comfortable with these choices. Finally, in some cases, patients may only want to eat foods of a certain color such as white foods or foods made from a single ingredient (e.g., apples). If this is the case, the nurse should try to provide these items initially so that the patient gets some nutrition. Eating issues often resolve as the patient's condition improves, and a few days of a fruit-only diet should not seriously harm most patients (although, of course, the nurse will want to bring this to the physician's attention).

The third type of intervention is *modifying the environment while reducing demands.* Family members can be helpful by bringing in preferred food or helping to get the patient to eat. The nurse can advocate for flexible visiting times for the patient to meet this need. The nurse may allow the patient to eat in her room if that is helpful to the patient. Finally, the unit schedule could be modified so that the patient can have access to food and fluids whenever they are willing to eat rather than waiting for scheduled meal times.

Help the patient take needed medications and cooperate with medical interventions. First, the nurse will want to *provide a rationale and offer verbal reassurance.* Medications pose a specific challenge, as they can be perceived as nonbeneficial or even poisonous. The nurse should always tell the patient what medication she is administering. For a paranoid patient, seeing the medication opened and/or looking at the medication administration record or medication packaging may be reassuring.

For the patient who becomes alarmed at a dosage change or a change in the appearance of the pill, calmly explaining the reason for the change can be helpful. Sometimes, explaining the purpose of medication can also help. For example, the nurse might say, "I know you are having a lot of trouble trusting anyone right now. You must feel very uncomfortable and afraid. I really believe that this medication will help you feel more comfortable."

It may take some time for the nurse using verbal reassurance to help the patient be able to take needed medications, but the nurse must consider that engaging in a power struggle with the patient (e.g., by insisting that the patient take the medications) runs the risk of ending in loss of trust and possibly in a restraint or seclusion. Consider the example of the paranoid patient who notices that her medications have changed. The nurse has brought the unopened pills and the medication administration record to administer the medications. The patient sees that the medication has changed, panics, grabs the pills, and refuses to give them back to the nurse. In this instance, the nurse administering the medication should remain calm and unrushed, and take his time in trying to reassure the patient rather than restraining her to retrieve the medications. The nurse may say, "We are giving you the correct medication." He may offer choices by saying, "You can keep that one or take it, or you can give it back to me and I will put it in a safe place." Finally, the nurse may offer explanations, such as "The doctor changed this because…" or "You take this because…"

In the extreme event that an injection must be given, consistency, clear explanations about the procedure, and verbal reassurance remain very important. The nurse should explain what she is doing and what medication she is giving to the patient. The nurse should provide verbal reassurance by saying, "I am giving you an injection of…this will help you feel calmer, less afraid…" The nurse can also say, "I know that you are afraid to take this, but we are going to watch you closely and make sure that you are okay." In most circumstances, these explanations are important to give, even if the nurse is not sure that the patient can understand them.

Second, the nurse will want to *offer choices*. Regarding medications, it may be beneficial for the nurse to acknowledge that the patient can refuse medication. "You can refuse to take this now. Do you want some time to think about it? I think it will help you. I can come back later and we can talk about this again." Alternatively, the nurse can say something like, "What if you choose one of these medications to take right now, and then take the other one in a little while?"

Third, with respect to *modifying the environment and reducing demands*, we note that there are fewer ways that the environment can be modified to encourage appropriate medication use. However, reducing demands is extremely important. With regard to medications, the nurse will decide how many medications to offer at a time, which ones to offer first, and how often to approach the patient about medications. For example, offering one medication at a time may be less overwhelming or anxiety provoking; however, one must also be careful about not approaching a patient too frequently, as this could also increase agitation.

Reducing demands is important to consider when other types of medical treatment are needed as well. Together with the rest of the treatment team, the nurse must weigh the urgency of the medical treatment and the difficulty it will pose for the patient. Consider the patient with diabetes who is refusing lab work or finger stick glucose checks or the patient with hypertension who is refusing to take medications or allow the nurse to monitor vital signs. The nurse may choose to have a discussion with the treating physician about whether they can wait a day or two to see if staff can develop more trust with the patient before insisting on these medical interventions. The team may decide that placing fewer demands initially on the patient is relatively safe and may help engage the patient in the end.

Intervene regarding poor hygiene. Again, the nurse will want to *provide a rationale and offer reassurance.* The nurse may say to the patient, "We think it is important that you do shower and get cleaned up because it will help you feel better...." The nurse can address any particular concerns the patient may have about the shower or bathroom. For example, he can put his own hands in the water to demonstrate that it is safe, or the nurse can offer to sit or have another trusted staff member sit outside the patient's bathroom while the patient showers. If the patient has a particular condition that makes hygiene very important, such as the patient's skin is at risk for breakdown, she is incontinent, or she has a condition, such as scabies or lice, that requires treatment, the nurse should clearly explain this to the patient.

There may also be ways that the nurse can *offer choices* or *reduce demands.* If a patient does not have a serious condition that requires bathing, bathing may not need to be a high-priority request, particularly for the first few days of treatment. The nurse can then offer choices like "Would you like to shower today, or just change your clothes?" or "Would you like to shower today or tomorrow?" The decision to give the patient these choices should be made in consultation with the treatment team.

STABILIZATION

● Subgoal: Decrease Fear and Anxiety

Fear and anxiety may underlie many of the patient's aggressive behaviors. Therefore, when the nurse is assessing risk for aggression or self-harm, as described previously, the nurse is also assessing underlying fear and anxiety. Individuals who have paranoid thoughts and feelings may also exhibit fear and anxiety without being at high risk for aggression (Herzog & Varcarolis, 2010; Williams, 1990). There are certain specific situations that may reliably lead to increased fear and anxiety in a patient with paranoia. These include having a roommate, visiting hours with the corresponding increased levels of noise and activity, other patients going into crisis, upcoming family meetings or discharge, inadvertent territorial violations, changes in the patient population such as admissions and discharges, and changes in staff.

Assessment of Fear and Anxiety

In report. In order to understand the patient's underlying level of fear and anxiety, the nurse will ask other staff if they have noticed any changes in levels of agitation. If the staff report that the patient has shown signs of increased anxiety, it is important to ask if staff have noticed any specific environmental or internal triggers.

One-to-one contact. The one-to-one conversation offers the nurse an opportunity to ask many specific questions.

Questions one might ask include "Is there a time you feel more worried?" "Is there any time you don't feel afraid?" "Are there certain things that make you feel more nervous or anxious about being here?" The nurse could also simply say, "Tell me what is going on." Any of these questions or comments may lead to insight about specific triggers or activities that might increase the patient's anxiety and fear. It may also be a good time to share any observations: "I notice you seem less anxious when the unit is quiet" or "I noticed you seem to be out of your room more. Are you feeling more comfortable here? Do you know what is helping you?"

The one-to-one interview will also provide an opportunity for the nurse to assess the patient's readiness for education about fear and anxiety. Is the patient beginning to demonstrate any insight to the linkage between fear, anxiety, and paranoia and the environment around him or her? Questions to ask the patient may include "What do you notice is happening around you when you have those thoughts?" or "Do you notice any triggers?" The nurse will watch for abrupt termination of the conversation or increased agitation, as these can indicate that the patient is not able to tolerate that level of discussion.

On the unit. As described previously, the nurse will want to assess nonverbal cues, such as psychomotor agitation, glaring, darting eye contact, and visual scanning, as these cues may indicate acute fear. The nurse will want to observe how much time the patient spends in his room, where he sits on the unit, and whether he joins others for group or meals. These observations give the nurse an indication of how comfortable the patient is in social situations.

● Key Nursing Interventions to Decrease Fear and Anxiety

Be aware of one's own nonverbal behavior, expressed emotions, and tone of voice. Particularly for the patient with paranoia, the nurse's nonverbal behaviors could influence the outcome of any intervention. Therefore, the nurse must be aware of her body language and posture, eye contact, and physical positioning when interacting with the patient. For example, it is helpful to avoid direct eye contact as this may be interpreted by the patient as a challenge. Sitting off to the side is less confrontational than sitting face to face, and this may decrease the patient's fear of being trapped. A nurse may choose to remain at the same physical level as the patient (i.e., if the patient is sitting, then the nurse should be sitting) or to assume a less threatening position by sitting down if the patient is standing up. A neutral stance, including keeping one's hands in view and not placing them behind the back or in pockets, will decrease the possibility of the patient perceiving the nurse as devious or hiding something.

Regarding expression of emotion, the nurse should keep in mind that nervous laughter or attempts to joke that may work with other patients can backfire with this individual. The patient who is paranoid may interpret these emotional expressions in unexpected ways and excessive smiling or laughing may be frightening. Alternatively, the patient may misinterpret jokes and kidding as ridicule; this will erode the trust the nurse is trying to develop. Therefore, the nurse will want to speak in a soft, calm tone whenever possible.

Provide verbal reassurance. The patient who is feeling fearful or afraid requires calm reassurance of their safety. Even if a patient is yelling, the nurse can choose to respond to the underlying emotion (fear) instead of the behavior or the paranoid cognitions. This allows the nurse to be reassuring and validating rather than confrontational or dismissive. For example, instead of saying, "Please do not yell out on the unit," the nurse may say, "We do not want to hurt you...you are safe, no one will harm you." Alternatively, after acknowledging the patient's fear, the nurse may try to ground the patient in reality by defining roles or routines: "We know you do not feel safe here...you do not know who to trust....but we are nurses and professionals and we want to help you." The nurse may also remind the patient of what the nurse is doing: "We are checking on you and the other patients so we can make sure you are okay...."

Treat the patient with respect. There are many ways in which the nurse conveys respect. Particularly with the patient with paranoia, answering questions truthfully and seriously addressing any concerns that the patient has helps to build the therapeutic alliance and trust. This may also reduce the patient's anxiety and fear if he feels that the nurse is listening to and understanding what is troubling him. Truthful answers can be reassuring to the individual who feels that everyone is lying and plotting to trick him. Respecting a patient's need for space or tolerance for interpersonal interactions also conveys respect in that the nurse demonstrates that she understands and values the patient's feelings. This can reduce anxiety and fear. If the patient is becoming more upset during a conversation, the nurse may try to end it as graciously as possible by saying something like "You seem to be getting more upset. I am going to give you some space" or "I am going to leave now and will be available at a later time...."

Finally, the nurse must convey respect for the patient's feelings while understanding and acknowledging that he does not agree with the patient's beliefs or delusions. It is not necessary to accept the person's paranoid delusions; however, it is also not useful to be dismissive or confrontational even if it feels therapeutic to the nurse. Being confrontational can often result in unproductive power struggles; therefore, the nurse should try to validate something in what the patient is saying. For example, if the patient believes that there are cameras in her room, the nurse can say, "I can see why you might think that the lights look like cameras, but I assure you there are no cameras, as it would not be allowed or even legal." As another example, a patient might state "I have to leave now. The police are coming to arrest me." The nurse can respond by saying: "I understand that it can be really hard to be here. I know you believe that the police are coming to arrest you. It must be awful to feel so afraid. However, I really do not think that they are coming and I want you to know that you are safe with us." Because it can be futile to try to reason or argue with a patient about their paranoid beliefs, the nurse may make one simple statement about reality and then change the subject. The nurse should not continue to disagree with the patient's beliefs. Instead, the nurse may encourage the patient to discuss other topics with a basis in reality, such as home life, work, school, and so on (Farhall, Greenwood, & Jackson, 2007).

Maintain consistency. If consistent staff is available, then the nurse should try to provide a consistent person to interact with the patient. New people may serve to increase anxiety substantially for this patient. Further, the nurse may want to try to minimize the room changes for this patient as this may trigger anxiety as well. The patient may not be able to accept or understand the rationale for room changes. If a room change is unavoidable, the nurse should consider whether there is someone already on the unit that would be a "good match" for this person before putting the paranoid patient in a room with a newly admitted patient.

Offer prn medications. Particularly, if the nurse can anticipate that an anxiety trigger, such as visiting hours, is forthcoming, the nurse may offer a prn medication such as a benzodiazepine.

Help the patient to identify soothing activities. Again, this may be particularly useful when the nurse can identify a trigger and then help the patient to prepare. Soothing activities include listening to music, being in the sensory room, and drawing or working on a craft project, depending on the patient's preference.

Take care in choosing roommates. The nurse can help the paranoid patient who may be able to have a roommate to be more successful if the nurse can choose someone who will be a "good fit." In general, the nurse will want to avoid having the potential roommate be someone who is on close observation or special or suicide precautions, as this would impose environmental restrictions and stressors on the person with paranoia. The nurse may also want to avoid assigning this patient a roommate who is actively self-injuring, manic, intrusive, or disorganized. The patient who is self-injurious or has manic behaviors may be too stimulating to someone with paranoia, who is having difficulty accurately interpreting the behavior of others. The individual who is intrusive will not be able to give this patient the space that he needs to feel less fearful or anxious. Finally, the patient who is disorganized, and in particular one who may be confused enough to take this patient's belongings, will only perpetuate the patient's fears of being preyed upon.

Be aware of what will not decrease fear and anxiety. It is unreasonable to expect that imposing behavioral consequences will diminish paranoid thoughts, beliefs, or behaviors. Consider the patient who is disruptive and yelling at other patients and staff. If the nurse tries to impose behavioral consequences such as making the patient go to her room or restricting the patient's privileges, then the patient will continue to feel afraid in addition to feeling punished or misunderstood. If the patient feels misunderstood, the therapeutic alliance may be damaged. Consequently, it may become more difficult to get the patient to take medications or try alternatives to calm her.

TREATMENT ENGAGEMENT

● **Subgoal: Increase Engagement in Inpatient Treatment**

Assess Willingness and Ability to Engage in Treatment on the Unit

As the fear and anxiety experienced by a patient with paranoia decreases and paranoid behavior is reduced, the patient's ability to engage in treatment should increase. In order to assess degree of treatment engagement in the unit, the questions that the nurse should keep in mind include "Is the patient taking medicine more easily?" "Is he participating in activities of daily living with less encouragement?" "How much time is the patient spending out of his room?" "Is he spontaneously socializing even a little?" "Is he out on the milieu more frequently, eating meals with others, and attending any groups?"

It is important for the nurse to keep in mind the individualized nature of paranoia and understand that each patient will demonstrate a different level of engagement on the unit. Some patients may be able to increase their treatment engagement a great deal as time on the unit passes; others may be able to take only small steps. In addition, the ability to tolerate other people or new activities may ebb and flow depending upon how the patient processes the experience. This is a situation where "one size does not fit all" and the nurse must determine the patient's ability to engage in treatment activities in the context of the patient's history and current activity levels. The nurse will want to assess and reassess treatment engagement on a regular basis using all sources of data, including information communicated in report, direct observation, and comments from the patient or family members. Combining the information received from these many sources will ensure that small improvements are noted and encouraged. This will also allow the nurse to determine what the next small step in treatment engagement might be for a particular patient and to encourage that step.

● Key Nursing Interventions to Increase Engagement in Treatment

When used successfully, all of the previously described interventions can help to engage the patient in treatment. Whenever the nurse is able to help the patient feel more comfortable in the hospital, assist the patient in getting a need met, or show respect for personal boundaries, the patient's fear and anxiety may decrease and the therapeutic alliance is strengthened. In addition, whenever the nurse successfully avoids a seclusion episode with this patient or succeeds in getting her to take medications, then engagement in treatment has begun.

Finally, when the nurse acknowledges the patient's feelings, approaches the patient without fear despite being rejected, and gives the patient choices, the nurse fosters trust, decreases fear and anxiety, and increases the likelihood that the patient will engage further in treatment. Encouragement to engage in treatment may increase as the patient progresses; in a stepwise fashion, the nurse may increase demands on the patient. This allows the patient to build on his or her previous success. In many cases, the nurse may not need to encourage the patient to engage further in treatment. Some patients will begin to approach staff more, eat, tend to their hygiene, take medications, and go to groups independently as symptoms improve.

Help to increase willingness to take medications. Since paranoid behaviors are symptoms of an underlying disease, one of the most important interventions will be to help the patient to take their antipsychotic medications. (See above sections and Chapter 12 for specific suggestions on how to do this.) Once the patient is taking medications, the nurse may have an opportunity to expand on medication teaching or assessment of the patient's ability to take medications independently.

Promote engagement in groups. Expecting a patient with paranoia to participate in all group activity or socialization opportunities is unrealistic. Even with some resolution of symptoms, some individuals will not be able to tolerate all of the activity on an inpatient unit. The nurse may see the opportunity to increase demands on the patient by inviting her to a group that she can tolerate. Better groups may be ones that include an individual activity (such as a craft) versus an open group discussion, more active groups (e.g., taking a walk), smaller groups, or groups that are not held in small enclosed rooms.

Encourage engagement in unit activities. As the patient's fear and anxiety decrease, the nurse may gradually increase demands on the patient by encouraging him to engage more in the community. For example, the nurse may invite the patient to eat outside of his room or to come to choose a meal as opposed to bringing food to the patient or letting the patient eat in his room. For example, in order to encourage engagement, the nurse may say, "We are having (insert dinner item) for dinner, why don't you come out and join us?" or "Come with me and see what is for lunch."

DISCHARGE PLANNING

Medication is the hallmark of treatment for the patient with paranoia. Therefore, educating the patient about medications, helping the patient consider the risks and benefits of medication adherence, and managing a medication schedule are important discharge considerations. There is a small percentage of patients for whom medication adherence will always be a struggle, and these patients may leave the hospital on long-acting injectable medications or court-ordered medications and outpatient treatment. The nurse's role in this case is to continue to be therapeutic with the patient. The nurse can acknowledge with him the difficulties he has in accepting medication or treatment. The nurse may be able to talk with the patient to elicit some benefits to taking medications. The nurse can share his own observations of improvement over the course of the hospitalization and how this is likely related to medications. The nurse should be honest and genuine in comments made about improvement in the patient's appearance, hygiene, nutrition, or ability to engage with others.

Finally, the nurse may want to discuss with the patient any fears related to the patient's residence or home environment. If the patient continues to have some fears but recognizes these as unrealistic, the nurse and the patient can discuss how the patient can reassure himself or from whom he can seek reassurance after discharge.

TABLE 7.1
Goals, Areas of Assessment, and Interventions for a
Patient With Paranoia

Goal	Assessment	Intervention
Safety		
Prevent aggression toward others	Understand recent history of aggression Look for problems with impulse control Observe patient's response to interactions Watch for obvious and subtle indicators of agitation Assess content of hallucinations or delusions	Offer verbal reassurance Modify the environment and reduce demands Provide sensory interventions Provide space and privacy Offer prn medication Use containment as a last resort
Prevent active self-harm	Remember this can be difficult to predict for these patients Understand history of self-harm Assess content of hallucinations or delusions Watch for agitation or isolative behaviors on the unit	Administer medications Increase monitoring Modify the environment Use containment as a last resort
Prevent passive self-harm	Monitor eating, output, weight, hygiene, and acceptance of needed medications or medical interventions	Provide a clear rationale and offer reassurance Offer choices Modify environment while reducing demands
Stabilization		
Decrease fear and anxiety	Assess agitation and look for environmental or internal triggers for anxiety Ask the patient directly about fear and anxiety Assess readiness for education about fear and anxiety	Be aware of one's own nonverbal behavior, expressed emotions, and tone of voice Provide verbal reassurance Treat the patient with respect Maintain consistency Offer prn medications

(cont.)

TABLE 7.1
Goals, Areas of Assessment, and Interventions for a
Patient With Paranoia *(cont.)*

Goal	Assessment	Intervention
Stabilization		
	Observe level of comfort in social situations	Help the patient to identify soothing activities Take care in choosing roommates
Treatment Engagement		
Increase engagement in inpatient treatment	Assess ability to accept medications, participate in activities of daily living, socialize, and attend groups Look for small improvements	Help to increase willingness to take medications Promote engagement in groups Encourage engagement in unit activities

REFERENCES

American Psychiatric Association. (2005). *Diagnostic and statistical manual of mental disorders*, 4th ed., text revision. Arlington, VA: Author.

Braham, I. G., Trower, P., & Birchwood, M. (2004). Acting on command hallucinations and dangerous behavior: A critique of the major findings in the last decade. *Clinical Psychology Review, 24*, 513–528.

Delaney, K. R., & Johnson, M. E. (2006). Keeping the unit safe: Mapping psychiatric nursing skills. *Journal of the American Psychiatric Nurses Association, 12*(4) 198–207.

Farhall, J., Greenwood, K. M., & Jackson, H. J. (2007). Coping with hallucinated voices in schizophrenia: A review of self-initiated strategies and therapeutic interventions. *Clinical Psychology Review, 27*(4): 476–493.

Favazza, A. R., & Rosenthal, R. J. (1993). Diagnostic issues in self-mutilation. *Hospital and Community Psychiatry, 4492*, 134–140.

Herzog, E. A., & Varcarolis, E. M. (2010). Schizophrenia. In E. A. Varcarolis & M. J. Halter, (Eds.), *Foundations of psychiatric mental health nursing: A clinical approach* (pp. 306–341). St. Louis, MO: Saunders.

Johnson, M.E. & Delaney, K.R. (2007). Keeping the unit safe: the anatomy of escalation. *Journal of the American Psychiatric Nurses Association, 13*(1). 42–52.

Krakowski, M. I., Czobor, P., Citrome, L., Bark, N., & Cooper, T. (2006). Atypical antipsychotic agents in the treatment of violent patients with schizophrenia and schizoaffective disorder. *Archives of General Psychiatry, 63*, 622–629.

Murphy, L., & Carson, E.B. (2010). Anger, aggression, and violence. In E. A. Varcarolis & M. J. Halter, (Eds.), *Foundations of psychiatric mental health nursing: A clinical approach* (pp. 565–583). St. Louis, MO: Saunders.

Quanbeck, C. (2006). Forensic psychiatric aspects of inpatient violence. *Psychiatric Clinics of North America, 29*, 743–760.

Quanbeck, C. D., & Mcdermott, B. E. (2008). Inpatient settings. In R. I. Simon & K. Tandiff, (Eds.), *Textbook of violence assessment and management* (pp. 259–276). Arlington, VA: American Psychiatric Publishing.

Schultz, S. H., North, S. W., & Shields, C. G. (2007). Schizophrenia: A review. *American Family Physician, 75*(12), 1821–1829.

Williams, D. (1990). Nursing care of the paranoid patient. *Advancing Clinical Care, 5*(6), 12–14.

Yearwood, M. S., & Shoemaker, N. C. (2010). Suicide. In E. A. Varcarolis & M. J. Halter, (Eds.), *Foundations of psychiatric mental health nursing: a clinical approach* (pp. 547–564). St. Louis, MO: Saunders

The Patient With Substance Use Disorders

8

Kristi Svendsen, Mary E. Dubreuil,
and Linda Damon

BACKGROUND AND DESCRIPTION

There are a variety of overlapping labels used to describe problems with substance use, including alcoholism, addiction, substance dependence, substance abuse, substance misuse, and hazardous substance use. In this chapter, we primarily use the terms *substance use disorders* and *substance dependence*. "Substance use disorders" is a broad term referring to substance dependence and abuse. Substance dependence is defined in the *Diagnostic and Statistical Manual of Mental Disorders, Fourth Edition, Text Revision* (APA, 2011) as the presence of at least three of the following symptoms within a 12-month period:

- Tolerance, as indicated by the need for a markedly increased amount of the substance to achieve the desired effect or a markedly diminished effect with continued use of the same amount of the substance;
- Withdrawal symptoms or use of the substance to avoid withdrawal symptoms;
- Greater intake of the substance or use over a longer period of time than intended;
- A persistent desire or unsuccessful attempts to cut down on substance use;

- A great deal of time spent on activities related to obtaining the substance, using the substance, or recovering from its effects;
- Giving up or reducing important social, occupational, or recreational activities because of substance use;
- Continued use of the substance despite knowledge of its having persistent negative physiological or psychological effects.

As can be seen from this definition, substance dependence is a complex phenomenon involving biological, psychological, social, and spiritual aspects of a person. Not all individuals with substance dependence experience all symptoms, but for many, substance dependence affects multiple domains of their lives.

This chapter will cover the process of detoxification and some of the problems associated with substance dependence that may be addressed within the short stay (e.g., 3–5 days) in a hospital setting. We note that dependence upon substances such as alcohol, benzodiazepines (e.g., clonazepam, alprazolam, or diazepam), and opiates/narcotics (e.g., oxycodone or heroin) will often involve withdrawal. In contrast, when people stop using cocaine or amphetamines, they do not experience such severe withdrawal symptoms.

Behavior

Patients who struggle with substance use disorders and seek treatment may present in very different ways.

- Some patients may freely acknowledge that they have a substance use problem and may be pleasant and cooperative and appear motivated for treatment and recovery.
- Other patients may not consider their substance use to be a problem. They may present in a guarded and

sometimes hostile manner. Such patients may come for treatment only because they have been told by a judge, spouse, or employer that they must seek treatment or they will lose their freedom, spouse, or job.

- Comorbid psychiatric disorders may affect patients' behavioral presentation. Depressed patients may be withdrawn, tearful, and minimally interactive. Others, who are in a manic phase of bipolar disorder, for example, may be hyperactive, irritable, loud, and demanding.
- Some patients are intoxicated when they arrive at the hospital and may be boisterous, belligerent, or extremely sedate and at risk for falling.
- Other patients may behave in secretive ways, whispering to other patients and potentially planning to bring contraband to the unit.
- Most patients with substance use disorders seek out nursing staff frequently, requesting medications to ease their anxiety.

Cognition

Patients with substance use disorders enter inpatient treatment with a variety of beliefs about the causes of their problems.

- Some patients come to treatment because they realize they have a problem and want help. They understand that, if not treated, their substance use may destroy them and cause devastating problems for their families. These patients may be eager to participate in treatment.
- Patients who come to the hospital for detoxification and treatment because somebody else has given them an ultimatum may think that the "other" person is the one with "the problem." Such thinking makes it difficult for patients to benefit from treatment, as they do not believe that their own thinking and behaviors need to

change. These patients may view treatment as an insult or an imposition.

- Other patients may think they are responsible for *having* a substance use disorder and may feel overwhelmed with guilt. These patients, especially those who keep relapsing and therefore need to repeat treatment, may think they are worthless and that their family members may be better off without them. Such patients may be contemplating suicide.
- Some patients may alternate between different types of cognitions. They may be torn between their desire to get well and the physical and psychological *need* to use. Many think, perhaps wishfully so, that they can learn to use in moderation.

Affect

Substance dependent patients going through detoxification on an inpatient unit may experience a variety of emotions, including the following:

- *Anxiety.* Some anxiety is a natural part of the physiological process of detoxification. Additional anxiety is often experienced because patients have difficult feelings and are unable to use their usual coping mechanism, that is, substances.
- *Shame.* Because of the stigma regarding substance dependence, many patients will feel ashamed. While this may be healthy at times and lead to positive changes, excessive shame can be very destructive for patients who are trying to recover.
- *Sadness.* While going through detoxification, many patients must face the losses that often accompany substance dependence, including loss of custody of children, marriage, job, or place of living. Many patients have serious medical consequences such as HIV, hepatitis C, and cirrhosis. Such losses also cause many patients to feel profound sadness and remorse.

- *Irritability.* Patients who do not believe they have a problem with substances and are being treated against their will may be irritable and express anger toward nursing staff.
- *Relief.* A few patients may express feelings of relief because they have made the decision to obtain treatment. Such patients may appear bright and hopeful.

Context

Many patients with substance use disorder have co-occurring illnesses, such as bipolar disorder, depression, mania, anxiety, obsessive–compulsive disorder, posttraumatic stress disorder, and chronic pain. The relationships between substance use and these disorders are often complex.

- Sometimes, a medical problem precedes the development of a substance use disorder. For example, patients who use opiates as prescribed for pain after surgery may become dependent and start to abuse the opiates and continue to have them prescribed after they no longer experience acute pain.
- Other patients have chronic pain. Learning to manage chronic pain with opiates without abusing them can be a daunting task for someone who has a substance use disorder. It may benefit such patients to find alternative ways to manage their pain. They could use anti-inflammatory drugs like ibuprofen or other nonaddictive pain relievers or they could benefit from another person holding and dispensing the prescribed opiates to them. Many patients who have never abused opiates have simply become physiologically dependent on the prescribed opiate they have been using for pain. When the source of their pain is no longer present, these patients, once detoxified, most likely will not experience the same psychological urge to continue to use opiates which typically afflicts patients with a substance use disorder.

- Often, people develop substance use disorder when they have been attempting to "medicate" underlying psychiatric disorders with alcohol or other drugs. Persons with bipolar disorder, for example, may have discovered that alcohol or other drugs help them cope with their extreme emotional ups and downs. Their drug use masks their underlying psychiatric illness which may be left untreated for years.
- In contrast, sometimes co-occurring illnesses, such as depression and anxiety, may be consequences of a substance use disorder. In such cases depression and anxiety may improve when the person is no longer using substances. In other cases, however, even if the depression or anxiety started after the abuse of substances, it may not improve even when the individual has stopped abusing substances.

POTENTIAL BARRIERS TO BEING THERAPEUTIC

Many people, including nursing staff, think of patients with substance use disorders as drug seeking, manipulative, hopeless, selfish, and lacking in the desire to change. This perspective makes engagement with the patient difficult, and the work can become unrewarding for the nurse. The nurse must challenge herself to reframe the way she is thinking about the patient's behavior. There are several types of beliefs that the nurse can reframe:

- *Seeing a patient as "med seeking."* Of course the patient is frequently requesting medications. This is the very way he has learned to cope when uncomfortable. The patient is probably not comfortable in the detoxification process.
- *Seeing a patient as "manipulative."* All human beings try to get their needs met, and if someone is not skilled in making direct requests, she finds other ways to try to get what she is looking for. Many times patients do not

have—and perhaps never learned—healthy communication skills.

- *Seeing a patient as "selfish."* Patients with substance use disorders require self-centered behavior to secure the drug, to justify the use of drug, to hide the behavior, and to push away the shame and guilt. People have to learn to consider others as they recover.
- *Seeing a patient as resistant to change.* What appears to be a lack of desire for change may in fact be fear of change or lack of necessary skills to change. If a person is on an inpatient unit, there is some part of her that desires change. If the nurse is with her in the process, there is always hope, always another opportunity for recovery.
- *Seeing a patient as "hopeless."* Change is a process that involves self-evaluation, experience, and development and practice of new life skills, among other things. It takes time to make a major life change, and few human beings do it perfectly the first time. If a person returns to treatment multiple times, the nurse can view this positively, as part of a process of learning and changing.

Reframing the patient's behavior and working from a positive perspective can help prevent the nurse from feeling frustrated and unrewarded.

OVERVIEW OF NURSING CARE GOALS

1. Safety
- Provide a *medically safe process of withdrawal* from substances
- Prevent contraband from being brought to the unit, and prevent "sharing" of prescribed medications between patients (diversion)
- Prevent suicide attempts and aggression

(continued)

OVERVIEW OF NURSING CARE GOALS (*continued*)

2. Stabilization
- Increase patient comfort during the withdrawal process
- Help patients begin to visualize a life without addicting substances

3. Engagement
- Assist patients by engaging in treatment on the unit

SAFETY

● **Subgoal: Provide a Medically Safe Process of Withdrawal From Substances**

Withdrawal from certain substances, particularly alcohol and benzodiazepines, may cause dangerous elevations in blood pressure for the first few days of withdrawal. If not treated, this may lead to seizures, strokes, or death. It is therefore crucial that vital signs and other indicators of withdrawal be monitored frequently for the first few days until vital signs are stabilized. For more information about the many possible medical complications associated with alcohol and benzodiazepine withdrawal, please refer McKeon, Frye, and Delanty (2008).

Withdrawal from opiates does not tend to produce great changes in vital signs, but the flu-like pain and discomfort of detoxification from opiates are often so distressing that patients are unable to tolerate this process without medical intervention.

Assessment of Risk for Potentially Life-Threatening Medical Complications Related to Detoxification

We recommend the use of a withdrawal assessment scale to measure the presence and intensity of withdrawal symptoms to ensure a medically safe detoxification process. The method used to assess and document withdrawal symptoms may vary from hospital to hospital. Such a withdrawal assessment document provides important information for all staff members about the detoxification process, including vital signs and other indicators of withdrawal. Based on this assessment, patients may then be medicated according to protocol. For an example, please see Figure 8.1.

In report. Report should include patients' recent vital signs, along with other symptoms of withdrawal, and a brief description of how patients seem to be tolerating the withdrawal process. If the patient is a new admission, report should include a history of not only psychiatric but also medical problems, especially those that may complicate withdrawal, such as hypertension or a seizure disorder. It is also important for nursing staff to know about any history of withdrawal seizures or delirium tremens. Other existing medical conditions to note are gastritis, bleeding, liver disease, heart disease, nutritional deficiencies, neurological impairment, and allergies, all of which may require changes to medications that are ordered routinely per protocol for symptoms of withdrawal.

One-to-one contact. The experience of withdrawal from alcohol and/or other substances varies from patient to patient. It is important that nursing staff consider both *subjective* symptoms (i.e., symptoms patients themselves report, like anxiety or headaches) and *objective* symptoms (i.e., symptoms which may be observed and measured, such as vital signs, tremors, sweats, chills, yawning, agitation or unsteady gait). With regard to subjective symptoms, patients' tolerance and perception of pain vary greatly. For this reason, some patients may become overmedicated and excessively sedate, while other patients may become undermedicated. With regard to objective symptoms, especially blood pressure and pulse, it is crucial that the nurse assesses vital signs every hour in patients with elevated

BIWA ORDER FORM

Allergies: _____ ☐ No known allergies

Name: _____

MR#: _____

Date	Time	ROUTINE ADMISSION ORDERS	Unit Clerk	Date time Posted/ Given	RN Signature
		If female (child bearing age) urine pregnancy test upon admission.			
		Breathalyzer & Urine toxicology screen upon admission and PRN for suspected substance use.			
		Vital Signs: BIWA scoring QID & PRN if BIWA>5 or P>110, SBP>150 or DBP>110.			
		Multivitamin w/Minerals 1 tab PO daily.			
		Folic Acid 1mg PO daily.			
		Thiamine 100mg PO on admission to unit and TID			
		PRN MEDICATION ORDERS			
		MD Initials — Dicyclomine 20mg PO Q6h PRN abdominal cramps. NTE 80 mg Q24h.			
		MD Initials — Bismuth Subsalicylate 30 ml PO Q2h PRN GI distress. NTE 120 ml Q24h.			
		MD Initials — Ibuprofen 400mg PO Q4h PRN for aches/pain NTE 2400mg Q24h.			

214

SUPPLEMENTAL ORDERS	Consider if the patient has one or more of the following: confusion, ataxia, visual complaints, malnourishment, chronic illness, elderly.		
	MD Initials	Thiamine 100mg IM upon admission to unit and TID x3 more doses.	
	MD Initials	Magnesium Sulfate 1gm IM upon admission	

BIWA MEDICATIONS (For Alcohol)

STANDARD PROTOCOL

	MD Initials	Lorazepam 1mg PO at 09:00 and 21:00 for 4 doses. Hold dose for sedation, If patient asleep or has nystagmus, or BAL>0.150.	
	MD Initials	Lorazepam 1mg PO Q1h PRN if BIWA>5, NTE 16mg Q24h. Hold dose for sedation, If patient asleep or has nystagmus, or BAL >0.150.	

CUSTOM PROTOCOL Consider if the patient has been consuming the equivalent of greater than 2 pints hard liquor, one case of beer, or high daily doses of sedatives.

	MD Initials	Lorazepam 2mg PO at 09:00 and 21:00 for 4 doses. Hold dose for sedation, If patient asleep or has nystagmus, or BAL >0.150.	
	MD Initials	Lorazepam 2mg PO Q1h PRN if BIWA>5, NTE 16mg Q24h. Hold dose for sedation, If patient asleep or has nystagmus, or BAL>0.150.	

BIWA MEDICATIONS (For Opiates)

	MD Initials	Lorazepam 0.5mg PO at 09:00 and 21:00 for 4 doses. Hold dose for sedation, If patient asleep or has nystagmus, or BAL >0.150.	
	MD Initials	Lorazepam 0.5mg PO Q1h PRN if BIWA>5, NTE 8mg Q24h. Hold dose for sedation, If patient asleep or has nystagmus, or BAL >0.150.	
	MD Initials	Clonidine 0.1mg PO at 09:00, 13:00, 17:00 and 21:00 for 8 doses. Hold if BP<90/50 or P<60 or for sedation.	

Signature: _____

❑ This page contains a Verbal Order

MR-1002 (1/2011)

FIGURE 8.1 Sample withdrawal assessment scale. (cont.)

BUTLER INSTRUMENT FOR WITHDRAWWAL ASSESSMENT
BIWA

BUTLER HOSPITAL Providence, Rhode Island Name: _____ MR#: _____

SCORES/Withdrawal Symptoms

- ☐ ETOH/SEDATIVES
- ☐ OPIATE/NARCOTIC
- ☐ BOTH SUBSTANCES

SCORES/Withdrawal Symptoms

SCORE 0-1: 0=NONE, 1=positive sx

SCORE 0-2: 0=NONE, 2=P > 100,
Systolic BP > or – to 150
Diastolic BP > or – tp 100

SCORE 0-3: 0=NONE, 1=mild,
2=moderate, 3=severe

BIWA Protocol/Special Consideration

*FOR MD CONSULT GUIDLINES (SEE BACK)

Start BIWA mediation:
If urine tox screen obtained,
BIWA >5, BAL <0.150 or
DR.'s order.

KEY
A = Alcolhol/Sedative wd.sx.
N = Opiate/Narcotic
A/N = Applied to Both

Please do not abbreviate
mediaction names

Date	Time	BP	P	T	R	0.2 PULSE > 100 SBP > 150 > 100	0-1 HEART RATE	0-1 TREMORS	0-1 PILOERECTION	0-1 YAWNING	0-1 CHILLS	0-1 PUPILS DILATED	0-3 AGITATION/ANXIETY	0-3 SWEATS/DIAPHORESIS	0-3 MUSCLE ACHES H/A	0-3 GI DISTURBACE	0-3 TREMOR	TOTAL SCORES	STAFF INITIALS	Comments
						A/N A/N	N	N	N	N	N	N	A/N	A/N A/N	A/N A/N	A/N	A A	A A		

WITHDRAWAL SYMPTOMS CATEGORIZED SCALE OF 1-3

ANXIETY/AGITATION:
1   Mild anxiety and observed increase in somewhat more than normal activity.
2   Moderately anxious, or moderately fidgety and restless.
3   Equivalent to acute panic states, or paces back and forth during most of the interview, constantly thrashes about.

PAROXYSMAL SWEAT:
1   Barely perceptible sweating, palms moist.
2   Beads of sweat observed on forehead
3   Drenching sweats.

GI DISTURBANCE:
1   Mild nausea with no vomiting or <3 incidents of diarrhea/24H.
2   Intermittent nausea with dry heaves or > 3 incidents of diarrhea/24H.
3   Constant nausea, frequent dry heaves, and vomiting or > 6 incidents of diarrhea.

TREMOR:
1   Not visible, but can be felt fingertip ti fingertip.
2   Moderate, while patient's arms extended.
3   Severe, even with arms not extended.

*CONSULT WITH MD:

If the patient has positive history of/or presents with current signs and symptoms of:

- DT's
- Withdrawal Seizure
- Hypertension
- Liver Disease, or is
- Allergic to a preprinted BIWA medication or
- Has persistent elevation in VS: Systolic BP > 200, Diastolic BP >110, P>120.

FIGURE 8.1 Sample Withdrawal Assessment Scale.

vital signs and look for any other signs of physiologic distress. In general, patients undergoing detoxification must be monitored for signs and symptoms of withdrawal at least every 4 hours.

On the unit. Nursing staff may also obtain important information about a patient's withdrawal process by observing behaviors on the unit when the patient may not know she is being observed. If a patient appears comfortable and is socializing with others, it may indicate fairly mild withdrawal symptoms. Sometimes, patients are unable to report symptoms to nursing staff, but may have observable symptoms such as sweating, disorientation, and sedation. Some individuals may display external signs that they are experiencing auditory or visual hallucinations, which could be indicative of alcoholic hallucinosis.

Although rare, patients who go through withdrawal from alcohol or benzodiazepines may develop delirium tremens. Such patients may become disoriented and may be observed wandering into other patients' rooms and lying down in other patients' beds. Their speech may become garbled, and they may experience drenching sweats and marked tremulousness. Some of these patients lose control over their muscles, becoming incontinent and unable to ambulate. Delirium tremens is a very serious medical condition. If changes in a patient's behavior suggest that he or she may be experiencing delirium tremens, such symptoms must be reported to the attending physician right away so that the physician may assess and direct further treatment.

Nursing staff may also observe another type of confusion in patients who are going through detoxification and being treated with benzodiazepines. After receiving repeated doses of benzodiazepines, some patients become disinhibited and disoriented, and they exhibit bizarre behaviors. Such symptoms, which may look very similar to intoxication from alcohol, must also be reported to the attending physician, who will assess and prescribe treatment for this condition. Behavioral disinhibition may look very similar to delirium tremens; however, it requires a very different treatment. Behavioral inhibition caused by "intoxication" from benzodiazepine treatment will require a reduction in benzodiazepine. On the other hand, delirium tremens, which usually causes an elevation of vital signs, will require an increase in the use of benzodiazepine.

● Key Nursing Interventions to Provide a Medically Safe Process of Withdrawal From Substances

Provide medication to stabilize vital signs. The most common medications used for patients withdrawing from alcohol or other drugs are benzodiazepines. Benzodiazepines are used to help reduce elevated vital signs, anxiety, and agitation.

Although withdrawal from opiates does not cause dangerous elevations of vital signs, patients who are being detoxified from opiates still tend to experience anxiety and agitation along with flu-like symptoms such as chills, body aches, and diarrhea. Clonidine, a medication that lowers blood pressure, is used because it has been found to significantly help reduce the painful symptoms associated with opiate detoxification, even though it is not needed to reduce blood pressure in these patients. For more information about the use of clonidine in opiate detoxification, see Polydorou and Kleber (2011).

For patients who are going through withdrawal from alcohol or benzodiazepines, and whose blood pressure remains dangerously high in spite of repeated doses of a benzodiazepine, the attending physician may prescribe clonidine to help reduce blood pressure.

Medications will be administered according to protocol for withdrawal symptoms as indicated by the results of the ongoing assessments (which should occur every 1–4 hours as per hospital protocol and as described above).

After a positive assessment for which patients receive a benzodiazepine and/or clonidine, they must be reassessed in 1 hour and medicated again, if indicated, then assessed again in another hour until vital signs and/or other signs of acute withdrawal subside. If blood pressure and/or pulse remain elevated in spite of repeated doses of medication according to protocol, it is important that the nurse consults the attending physician for additional orders for medications such as clonidine to help return the patient's vital signs to within safe parameters.

In cases where a patient becomes confused and may be developing delirium tremens (to be assessed by the attending physician), the physician will usually order increased amounts of benzodiazepines and sometimes neuroleptics (i.e., antipsychotic medications). For patients who become behaviorally disinhibited because they cannot tolerate the amount of benzodiazepine prescribed for their detoxification, the treatment will include a reduction in the use of benzodiazepines. Close monitoring and communication with the attending physician is important in managing these symptoms and differentiating between the two problems.

● **Subgoal: Prevent Contraband From Being Brought to the Unit and Prevent "Sharing" of Prescribed Medications Between Patients (Diversion)**

There is always a risk that patients who seek inpatient treatment for their substance dependence may try to bring alcohol or drugs (i.e., contraband) to the unit. Some may have contraband with them at time of admission. Other patients may arrange to have someone bring contraband to the unit after they have been admitted. Even if patients make the decision to stop using alcohol and/or other drugs and seek treatment, many patients experience strong urges to use their drug of choice, especially when they are going through the discomfort of withdrawal. Contraband is a safety issue because patients who use drugs in addition to those being prescribed for them on the unit put themselves at a great risk for an overdose. Contraband brought to the unit can endanger the life of any patient with whom it is shared.

Assessment of Signs of Contraband Being Brought to the Unit

In report. It is crucial that any unusual patient behaviors be discussed in report, especially secretive behaviors. In addition, nursing staff will want to know about any previous history of a patient bringing contraband to the unit.

One-to-one contact. Nursing staff may obtain information regarding contraband only indirectly by observation and by listening to patients. Sometimes, one patient will tell the nurse that another is making arrangements to have drugs brought to the unit or is sharing his prescribed medications. However, the nurse should not assume that all detoxing patients are planning to have contraband brought to the unit. If there is nothing indicating this possibility, nursing staff should not ask the patient if he has brought in contraband or if he is thinking about bringing contraband to the unit. If the nurse asks such questions without any evidence, the patient will likely feel unjustly accused.

On the unit. It is important for nursing staff to pay attention to changes in patients' behaviors as they interact with other patients on the unit. A patient who may be contemplating having contraband brought to the unit may be seen whispering to other patients, or may stop talking or become hostile when nursing staff come near her. Often such a patient will spend a lot of time on the phone and may try to involve other patients. It is also important to pay attention to visitors who try to visit away from the open areas of the unit and/or are hostile toward staff.

● Key Nursing Interventions to Prevent Contraband From Being Brought to the Unit

Search patients and their belongings. It is important that a very careful metal detection and pat search be performed on every patient upon admission and upon every return from pass, and that all patients' belongings are examined carefully before being given back to the patients. When additional belongings are brought in for patients after admission, such items also need to be carefully checked before they are given to patients. Potential ways patients may bring in pills include putting pills into a seam in a piece of clothing or taping pills to the body. Potential ways of bringing in alcohol include hiding a flask in a shirt pocket; this may not be detected if the pat search is superficial.

Educate and observe visitors. There is a risk for contraband being brought to the unit by "well-meaning" family members or friends. Therefore, nurses must ask all visitors if they are bringing in anything for the patients. All such items must be inspected before given to the patients. Visits should always take place in common areas, and not in patient rooms. Additional protocols regarding visitors vary by institution or agency. Depending on the facility's policy, visitors may not be pat searched, and the visitors' pockets and pocketbooks may not be checked. It can help to have educational groups for patients' family members and friends in order to help them better understand substance use disorders and help to counter a family member's belief that he is "helping" a patient by bringing in drugs. In particular, family members should understand that contraband could lead to overdose or dangerous drug–drug interactions.

Lead discussion about contraband in community groups. Another proactive way to help prevent drugs from being brought to the unit is to discuss the issue of contraband openly in community groups. Staff may talk in supportive ways about how normal it is for persons with substance use disorders to have urges to use, and may remind patients that such urges or cravings will pass. In community groups, patients may be encouraged to approach staff if they should feel such cravings. Staff may be able to help patients "talk through" such difficult moments. This may help reduce the likelihood that patients will attempt to bring in contraband.

In community groups, nursing staff may also ask all patients to alert staff if they become aware of safety issues on the unit such as the presence of contraband or patients sharing prescribed medications. In order to acknowledge that some patients may not want to "tell" on their peers, nursing staff should emphasize the fact that they are only interested in all patients' safety. In order to illustrate this point, a nurse may ask patients what they would do if they saw someone having a seizure on the unit. Most patients would respond that they would alert staff immediately. The nurse could then suggest that the presence of contraband on the unit is just as serious and potentially life threatening as a seizure may be.

Finally, in community groups, it is important to encourage patients to talk with each other about recovery and healthy behaviors, and to discourage talk about drug-using behaviors. Discussion about drug use may increase urges to use drugs and thoughts of trying to have contraband brought to the unit.

Provide stimulating activities for patients. Another proactive intervention is to keep the unit active with a variety of groups and other healthy activities available for patients. This will help patients stay focused on recovery and distract them from dwelling on past unhealthy behaviors.

Intervene if contraband is found or suspected. If drugs or paraphernalia are found on the unit or there is a marked change in a patient's mental status, the nurse must investigate immediately. This includes asking the patient directly if he has taken more medication than what is prescribed. This may be done in a nonjudgmental way by always emphasizing that patient safety is the issue. A nurse may say "I have noticed that you have become very sedate, and I am worried about this." The nurse may suggest checking vital signs and talk with the patient about the dangers of an overdose. Whether a patient admits to having brought in drugs or not, sudden increases in sedation need to be reported to the attending physician immediately. Sometimes, such unfortunate incidents may lead to life-threatening situations which could require emergency IV treatment.

● Subgoal: Prevent Suicide Attempts and Aggression

Some patients who are going through detoxification, and especially those with comorbid depression and/or bipolar disorder, may be at risk for committing suicide. These individuals must be closely monitored and assessed for suicide risk. Other patients who are going through detoxification may demonstrate irritability and aggressive behavior and may need assistance with anger management. We refer the readers to Chapter 9, "The Patient Who Is Suicidal," and Chapter 1, "The Patient With Anger," for details on how to manage these problems.

STABILIZATION

● Subgoal: Increase Patient Comfort During Withdrawal Process

Even when a patient is not experiencing withdrawal symptoms that indicate that she is in some type of physical danger, withdrawal can be very uncomfortable. Patients may experience insomnia, agitation, headaches, or other types of pain.

Assessment of Patient Discomfort During the Withdrawal Process

In report. In report, nursing staff may discuss how a patient seems to be managing without using substances. Is he able to sleep, eat, and participate within the unit milieu? Is he complaining of pain? Does he utilize available comfort measures, or does he need education or encouragement from nursing staff?

One-to-one contact. This may provide nursing staff with information about specific types of discomfort a patient is experiencing and potential barriers that keep the patient from taking advantage of available healthy ways to help herself feel better. Nurses should directly inquire about feelings of anxiety or pain and ask if the patient remembers how she handled anxious feelings before she began using addicting substances. To assess barriers to accessing comfort measures, a nurse may ask a patient, "So, what have you been doing to manage your headache?" "Has it worked?" "What would you like to try?" "Have you considered trying ibuprofen?" "If not, why?"

On the unit. Nursing staff may observe how patients are doing within the unit milieu. This may sometimes appear different from a patient's self-report. One patient may tell you that he is having trouble sleeping, but appear to be sleeping reasonably well on overnight shifts. Other patients may minimize discomfort, but actually appear to be in a fair amount of pain. Further, on the unit, nursing staff should look for ways in which a patient seeks to comfort or soothe herself. The nurse may discover that a patient has a particular strength (e.g., socializing with other patients). The nurse can then discuss that strength with a patient, including the ways in which it can be a source of comfort.

● **Key Nursing Interventions to Increase Patient Comfort During Withdrawal Process.**

Offer nonaddictive medications. It is very common for patients who struggle with addiction to request addictive medications (e.g., benzodiazepines or opiates) whenever they feel uncomfortable or upset. It is important to educate patients about the fact that many problems can be addressed with medications that are not addictive. For example, patients may receive Motrin or Tylenol for headaches or muscle aches. Bentyl may help patients who are experiencing stomach cramping. Initially, a patient may reject nonaddictive medications. A patient may require extra encouragement to try such medications and then to evaluate whether or not they are helpful.

Offer comfort measures. These might include a pitcher with ice water or juice (which may also help prevent dehydration), an extra blanket or soothing music from a CD player, showers, rest, music, a walk, and relaxation techniques. Many patients with substance use disorders seem to have "forgotten" the many, simple, healthy means of comfort that are readily available. Consistently offering these comfort measures on the unit will help teach patients to consider these alternatives in the future.

● **Subgoal: Help Patients Begin to Visualize a Life Without Addicting Substances**

Assessment of Readiness to Visualize a Life Without Addicting Substances and What That Life May Look Like

In report. Often, patients need to seek treatment several times before they begin to understand their illness and their own role in the recovery process. Recovery and healing involves a lot more than simply not using addictive substances. Report should include information about the patient's history of substance use disorders, what kinds of treatments he has tried in the past, and if such treatments have been helpful. Such information will give nursing staff some indication of what kind of plan for a life without substances might work for this particular patient. Some patients will arrive at the hospital with a plan for "aftercare" already in mind; others will not. For example, patients who have failed intensive outpatient treatments in the past may have decided that they need long-term residential treatment. Other patients may only want to attend Alcoholics Anonymous (AA) or Narcotics Anonymous (NA), and still others may want counseling. Some patients will need to see a psychiatrist regarding co-occurring disorders. Patients who suffer from chronic pain may want help finding out how they can safely manage chronic pain while minimizing the threat of relapse.

One-to-one contact. This will give the nurse an opportunity to assess where a patient is in terms of (1) readiness to accept treatment after admission, (2) readiness to consider a life without substances, and (3) plans for what such a life might look like. The nursing assessment can be particularly important because often patients agree to the doctor's suggestions for aftercare without thinking things through carefully. The nurse can help the patient to adopt an aftercare plan that is feasible and appropriate for her particular situation.

On the unit. By observing how patients interact with other patients on the unit, the nurse may see some clues about how ready the patient is to make major life changes, to stop using substances, and to accept treatment. Patients who tend to dwell on the past and discuss drug-using behaviors with other patients may need additional help in visualizing a future without addictive substances. In contrast, patients who talk about healthy activities they can start on the unit and what they plan to do after discharge are helping themselves and may also inspire other patients to do the same.

● **Key Nursing Interventions to Help Patients Visualize Their Lives Without Addicting Substances**

Provide education and opportunities to visualize a different type of life. Patients will often require direct teaching about what a life without addictive substances can look like. Many patients will benefit from being reminded of the importance of developing simple habits like eating a healthy diet and adding simple exercises like walking to their daily routine. A patient may also be encouraged to think about starting other healthy activities that he has enjoyed previously, such as playing an instrument, being involved in sports, journaling, taking part in religious activities, or volunteering. The nurse will want to encourage a patient to be as concrete and specific as possible as he thinks about how his life might be different. A simple group activity that may help patients visualize a healthy life is to ask patients to make a two-sided collage. On one side of a poster board, patients may glue pictures and words from magazines that describe their past. On the other side, patients may be asked to arrange pictures and words describing the future they are starting to visualize.

In addition to education regarding substance use disorders, patients also need education regarding healthy ways to cope with co-occurring psychiatric disorders, medical problems, and/or chronic pain.

Participation in support groups like AA or NA can be very helpful for patients. AA and NA commitment groups may come to the hospital to tell patients about their program. In such groups, patients may learn from the example of their peers who have come to live healthy, happy, and productive lives without addicting substances.

Help patients learn to manage their emotions. For most patients who have used alcohol and/or other drugs as a way to escape from difficult emotions, it is frightening to think about facing difficult emotional experiences without substances. Further, when patients come to the hospital for treatment, they often have to deal with very painful feelings of regret associated with the often devastating consequences of their addictive behaviors prior to treatment. Educational groups focusing on coping skills, emotional management, and anger management can be very helpful. It is also important for nursing staff to educate patients about the transitory and potentially adaptive nature of difficult emotions. Patients will benefit from learning (again) that feelings give people important information about themselves.

Patients who struggle with substance use disorders very often blame themselves for their illness. Patients may benefit from a nurse emphasizing that blaming (others or oneself) does not help the healing process, as it distracts patients from moving toward a new life. Nursing staff may help to reduce self-blame by educating patients about the biological basis for substance use disorders. A patient's genetic inheritance and early life experiences was and is not under the patient's control. Still, patients must understand that, like all persons who have an illness, they have responsibilities and choices regarding their healing process. This view may help to counter the stigma surrounding substance use disorders. It may also empower patients as they consider their paths of healing.

Help with goal setting. The nurse will work with the patient to help establish the patient's own personal goals for treatment. If the nurse enters this process with her own agenda, it will be more difficult to engage the patient in the process. Instead, the nurse should find out what is important to the patient, ask questions, and make suggestions about what the patient might consider in order to reach her identified goals. In the end, people work toward things they really desire and not what is imposed upon them. The nurse can act as a guide to help the patient discover what is really important to her, as opposed to forcing a situation in which the patient is trying to please treatment providers or significant others.

Educate family members. Families also need education and help in visualizing a life in which their loved one is not abusing substances. Such education may be done through individual family meetings or in group discussions where all patients and their family members may participate. Family members tend to experience a lot of emotional pain and confusion when a family member develops a substance use disorder. Often, the whole family becomes "sick" as they try to figure out how to interact with a family member with a substance use disorder. Family members may need to make changes, and they may also benefit from learning about AA or NA. These are community support groups for family members and friends of persons who struggle with addiction.

TREATMENT ENGAGEMENT

● **Subgoal: Assist Patients to Engage in Treatment on the Unit**

Assess Willingness and Ability to Engage in Treatment on the Unit

There are several factors that may impact an individual's ability to engage in treatment on the unit, including (1) the patient's reason for coming in for treatment, (2) the patient's "stage of change" (described below); (3) cognitive functioning; and (4) past treatment experience.

It is important for the nurse to understand precipitating factors leading a patient to seek treatment. Admission is a good time to ask a patient about this, as it is likely to be in the forefront of his mind at that time. Generally speaking, people move toward change when their behavior is negatively impacting their lives. Some people present with a better understanding of the negative consequences of their substance use and understand how they are responsible for the consequences. Others have an external locus of control and look outside themselves for explanations as to why they are using alcohol and drugs. However, each person has a bottom line reason for seeking treatment, one that is important to them. Understanding this reason may give the nurse a way to start engaging the patient in treatment.

Also important in being best able to engage the patient is to determine her readiness for change. Prochaska and DiClemente (1983, 1992) have identified the following "stages of change": precontemplation (not even considering making a behavior change), contemplation (considering change), preparation (getting ready to change), action (actually making behavior changes), and maintenance (maintaining new patterns of behavior). Each stage requires a different approach to engaging the patient. For example, if a person is in the contemplative stage and is approached by a member of the nursing staff who is enthusiastically trying to help her build a recovery plan, the nurse's efforts will most likely be met with either irritation or passive agreement. Neither response is an indicator that the patient is actively engaged in the process. When the nursing staff member is gone, most frequently, so is the plan. The nurse will want to repeatedly assess the patient's stage of change, as it is a dynamic process. Questions to ask to determine the stage of change might include the following:

- What brings you to the hospital today?
- What is it like for you to be on a detox unit?
- What are you most concerned about regarding your substance use?
- Many people feel anxious about giving up substances. What concerns you most about that?
- Not everyone who comes into the hospital has made a decision to be abstinent. Where are you in the process of making that decision for yourself?
- What do you see as the negative consequences of your substance use?
- How has your substance use impacted your life?

- What is it like to think about stopping the use of alcohol and/or drugs?
- Tell me a little about your family. What do they tell you about your substance use?
- What are your goals for this treatment?

The nurse should also be observing cognitive functioning, as this can impact treatment engagement. There are times when a patient is unable to fully engage in treatment because of the effects of medications or even brain damage due to long-term drug use. Although the nurse does not diagnose cognitive impairment, she will be in the position of observing the patient's functioning on the unit and reporting the observations to the physician. The nurse should carefully review admission assessments, including mental status exams, any prior psychological or neuropsychological testing, and any assessments done by the attending physician. Some of the ways a nurse might look for cognitive impairment is by observing the way the patient interacts with his environment and peers, whether he is able to remember past conversations, whether he is able to follow a topic in group or individual sessions, his ability to follow instructions, and his ability to participate in making a plan for his recovery. Understanding cognitive functioning is so important because trying to engage a person at a level at which he is unable to succeed is frustrating for the patient and for the nurse and may lead to a decrease in motivation, confidence, and self-esteem for both. Many cognitive deficits improve over time and with abstinence; however, nursing staff on a detoxification unit may not be witness to this part of the healing process.

Finally, the nurse should assess the patient for past experience with treatment and abstinence. As with any change process, experience is important. The more experience a person has with maintaining abstinence from alcohol and/or drugs, the more of a foundation there is for the person to build on. The nurse will want to gather evidence of successful treatment experiences in the past.

● **Key Nursing Interventions to Increase Engagement in Treatment**

Use motivational enhancement techniques. Nurses working with patients with substance use disorders have a role in helping the patient enhance their motivation for recovery. The nurse can help the patient move along the continuum of stages of change in a positive direction. In order to do so, a nurse should work to develop an empathic, patient, and curious attitude toward the patient and his experience with his illness, as well as a belief that human beings have the capacity to heal and grow. Once the nurse believes in the patient's ability to change, she can assist the patient in recognizing his strengths, which in turn can foster hope and optimism for the future.

If a person presents in a precontemplative phase of change, it is important for the nurse to take the time to connect with the patient in a nondirective way, in order to build rapport and trust. The nurse might engage the patient in a discussion about what brought him into treatment or help the person to explore the pros and cons of abstinence from alcohol and drugs. Nurses working on an inpatient detoxification unit are in a unique and critical position to effect a change in motivation, since motivation can be driven by the recognition of negative consequences. Rarely are negative consequences more acutely present in the minds of people with substance use disorders than when they are admitted to the hospital.

If the patient is in the contemplative phase, the nurse might want to normalize the patient's ambivalence about making changes in her life. This may help the patient to see the nurse as nonjudgmental and willing to help the patient make her own decision about recovery. In this way, the patient has more freedom to talk about her real feelings rather than what she thinks the nurse wants to hear. This is also an opportunity to help the patient identify personal values and determine how those values relate to the recovery process.

For the patient in the preparation phase of change, the nurse might ask the patient to identify personal goals and begin to help the patient put together a plan to achieve the goals. This plan might include helping the patient to eliminate any potential barriers to change, such as transportation or financial concerns.

Finally, for a patient who is actively in the process of changing her life, that is, in the action phase, the nurse might help the patient to identify triggers, thoughts, and feelings that precede the drinking or drugging behavior and to develop alternative coping strategies to deal with them. The nurse might also help the patient set small, achievable goals toward recovery.

Tailor interventions for patients with impaired cognitive functioning. This patient might be best served by engaging in a very concrete manner, assisting with structure, focus, and positive relationship building. The nurse should also let the patient know that some of the problems he is experiencing, such as memory problems and difficulty in concentrating, are normal in early recovery. Normalizing some of the cognitive difficulties can reduce fear and increase engagement.

Use past treatment experiences as important information. The nurse can help the patient see the value of past treatments and periods of abstinence for use in recovery and relapse prevention. Patients may minimize or disregard their own abilities, believing that any slip from abstinence erases past successes. Some community-support groups reinforce this type of thinking by having people set new abstinence anniversary dates for any slip. Engaging the patient in a discussion about past successes with abstinence, including what worked and what did not work, can help the person recognize her strengths and hold on to things that were helpful, while discovering areas that require new or additional strategies.

Build trust. A nurse must build a respectful, trusting relationship with the patient. When a patient is held in high regard and approached with respect, all else flows more smoothly. Few people are comfortable working with a health care professional with whom there is no rapport or who is experienced as emotionally disconnected or worse, judgmental. It is important to invest some time in getting to know the patient; finding out what is important to him is time well spent. Later on, it will be easier to ask difficult questions or to make recommendations the patient may not be inclined to embrace. To help build a therapeutic relationship, the nurse will always focus on listening to the patient. She will ask questions related to what she's hearing from the patient and be curious about him. The nurse will avoid confrontation, even if she believes that the patient is not facing the truth or not accepting responsibility for his behavior. When the nurse has engaged in this way with the patient, the patient will most likely be more willing to engage with the nurse.

Do not compel the use of labels, make assumptions, or force confrontations. It is important that the nurse not try to force the patient to label himself as an alcoholic or addict in order to move forward in the recovery process. In fact, this may create a more adversarial relationship with the nurse. Labels have the tendency to box people in and rob them of their individual differences. There is little room for the patient to discuss his situation in an authentic manner with the nurse. Assumptions made by the nurse that she "knows what the patient needs" are equally constricting to the development of a trusting relationship. Confrontation regarding any aspect of the patient's experience, if conducted in an intense or hostile manner, may result in conflict and opposition rather than a joining between nurse and patient. Even if the "challenge" is presented gently, the nurse should remember that any challenge should be delivered within the context of an already trusting relationship, and the nurse should begin by asking the patient's permission to point out her observation to him. The nurse should keep in mind that the ability to offer a challenge to a patient is an earned right that develops between the nurse and the patient.

Facilitate participation in group therapy. Group therapy has been found to be an effective treatment for people in recovery from addictive disorders (Brown & Yalom, 1977; Flores, 1997). Group allows the patient to identify with others, improve interpersonal communication, get feedback from peers, obtain important information, and develop new coping skills. Group can be intimidating for patients, so the nurse might begin by inviting the patient to sit in group without pressure to participate. Group can also be challenging for those who are feeling physically ill. In that case, the nurse can let the patient and the other group members know, in advance, that it is all right for the patient to excuse herself if she is not feeling well enough to continue.

Encourage engagement in unit activities. Activities are also important to the recovery process. The nurse can help the patient see how the activities fit in with the overall recovery plan and the development of healthy alternatives. For example, she might help the patient to see how unit activities are, in fact, an introduction to leisure skills. For many patients, leisure deficits and difficulty having fun without alcohol and drugs can lead to relapse. The patient might complain of too much free time and of feeling bored. The nurse can help the patient to find activities to do that are in line with his own goals and interests.

PREPARATION FOR DISCHARGE

Educate about medications and attitudes toward medications. Patients may hear conflicting opinions in the community regarding the use of medications. Nurses are in a great position to present objective data on the use of such medications as antabuse, suboxone, naltrexone, and various antidepressants. This will help patients prepare for possible opposing opinions that might be encountered outside of the hospital.

Help the patient anticipate challenges. The recovery process is rarely easy and often includes many difficult losses, including loss of the use of alcohol and drugs. Many times, patients can present in a way that appears to be the perfect example of recovery. If it looks too good to be true, it probably is. This is not to say that the nurse cannot celebrate successes and positive feelings with the patient, but to celebrate before exploring what is beneath the patient's enthusiastic and positive presentation might be a missed opportunity. The nurse must understand there is sometimes so much pain, shame, and guilt related to substance use that the patient may begin doing everything "right" as a way of avoiding the focus on a more painful past. The reality will eventually surface and the nurse can help the patient anticipate that possibility by acknowledging the patient's good work and by providing education about the normal ups and downs that occur in the process of recovery and what feelings might arise in the future. In this way, the nurse helps the patient anticipate and normalize difficulties that might come up after discharge.

Review aftercare plans. In reviewing aftercare plans, the nurse can make certain the patient is clear about the next step in the recovery process. He can answer any questions and address any unresolved concerns the patient may have about the level of care he has selected following discharge from the hospital. In addition, the nurse can help the patient outline the issues she has uncovered during the hospitalization that might require her additional attention after discharge.

TABLE 8.1
Goals, Areas of Assessment, and Interventions for a Patient With Substance Use Disorders

Goal	Assessment	Intervention
Safety		
Provide a medically safe process of withdrawal from substances	Obtain information about patient's history of complications during detoxification, including seizures and DTs Use a standardized detoxification assessment scale every 1 to 4 hours to obtain and record vital signs and other withdrawal symptoms	Provide medications to stabilize vital signs
Prevent contraband from being brought to unit and prevent "sharing" of prescribed medications between patients (diversion)	Obtain information about patient's history of bringing contraband to unit Listen to other patients who may provide information about contraband Observe sudden changes in mental status or sudden increase in sedation	Search patients and their belongings Educate and observe visitors Lead discussion about contraband in community groups Provide stimulating activities for patients Intervene if contraband is found or suspected
Prevent suicide attempts and aggression	Please see Chapter 9, "The Patient Who Is Suicidal" and Chapter 1, "The Patient With Anger"	
Stabilization		
Increase patient comfort during withdrawal process	Observe how each patient is functioning and assess level of comfort Observe patient's use of comfort measures	Offer nonaddictive medications Offer comfort measures

(cont.)

TABLE 8.1
Goals, Areas of Assessment, and Interventions for a Patient With
Substance Use Disorders (*cont.*)

Goal	Assessment	Intervention
Stabilization		
Help patients begin to visualize a life without addicting substances.	Assess readiness to visualize such a life Look for clues about what such a life would like for this particular patient	Provide education and opportunities to visualize a different type of life Help patients learn to manage their emotions Help with goal setting Educate family members
Treatment Engagement		
Assist patients to engage in treatment on the unit	Assess patient's reason for coming in for treatment, readiness to engage in treatment, cognitive functioning, and past treatment experience	Use motivational enhancement techniques Tailor interventions for patients with impaired cognitive functioning Use past treatment experiences as important information Build trust Do not compel the use of labels, make assumptions, or force confrontations Facilitate participation in group therapy Encourage engagement in unit activities

REFERENCES

American Psychiatric Association. (2011). *Diagnostic and statistical manual of mental disorders* (4th ed.). Arlington, VA: Author.

Brown, S., & Yalom, I. D. (1977). Interactional group therapy with alcoholics. *Journal of Studies on Alcohol, 30*(3), 426–456.

Flores, P. J. (1997). *Group psychotherapy with addicted populations: An integration of twelve-step and psychodynamic theory* (2nd ed.). New York: The Haworth Press.

McKeon, A., Frye, M. A., & Delanty, N. (2008). The alcohol withdrawal syndrome. *Journal of Neurology, Neurosurgery & Psychiatry, 79*, 854–862.

Polydorou, S., & Kleber, H. D. (2011). Detoxification of opioids. In M. Galanter & H. D. Kleber, (Eds.), *American psychiatric publishing textbook of substance abuse treatment* (pp. 265–287). Arlington, VA: American Psychiatric Publishing.

Prochaska, J. O., & DiClemente, C. C. (1983). Stages and processes of self-change of smoking: Toward an integrative model of change. *Journal of Consulting and Clinical Psychology, 51*, 390–395.

Prochaska, J. O., DiClemente, C. C., & Norcross, J. C. (1992). In search of how people change: Applications to addictive behavior. *American Psychologist, 47*, 1102.

The Patient Who Is Suicidal   9

Linda Espinosa, Angela Macera,
Elizabeth Harris, Barbara-Ann Bybel,
Judith L. Giorgi-Cipriano, and
Julie Armstrong Muth

BACKGROUND AND DESCRIPTION

Patients who suffer from a psychiatric illness are at increased risk for suicide. Those who are hospitalized for the treatment of a psychiatric illness because they are experiencing an acute exacerbation of their symptoms are at even higher risk (Munich & Greene, 2009, pp. 32–33). Therefore, assessment for suicide risk is necessary for every psychiatric inpatient at the time of admission and periodically throughout the course of their stay in the hospital.

Behavior

Longitudinal risk. Patients who are at risk for suicide may have different presentations. Many of these patients are visibly sad with a noticeable slowing down of their thinking, speech, and movements. Often they have difficulty sleeping, tending to awaken considerably earlier than they would like and failing to return to sleep. This loss of sleep often leads to an appearance and a feeling of extreme fatigue. They may lose their appetite, complaining that food is tasteless to them or lacks flavor. They may appear unkempt with a lack of attention to personal hygiene.

For a considerable number of patients at risk for suicide, their presentation is in some ways the opposite of the above. Instead of being unable to sleep, they may oversleep, remaining asleep in bed literally all day every day unless encouraged to get up. Rather than being slowed down physically, some may appear visibly agitated with pacing and wringing of the hands. Finally, instead of losing their appetite, some people overeat in an attempt to soothe themselves.

When patients are at risk for suicide as a result of psychotic symptoms, their appearance may be quite different. For example, a patient in a manic state may believe he can fly and may jump to his death from a bridge or high building. A patient who hears voices that command her to kill herself may behave in bizarre ways and attempt suicide in exactly the way the voices instruct.

Patients at risk for suicide may have poverty of speech, speaking only briefly when directly questioned. They may seem quite withdrawn and distant. When they do speak, it may be about death or suicide, or they may focus on physical symptoms making them miserable: constipation, headache, exhaustion, or back pain, for example.

Acute risk. Some specific behaviors are especially indicative of suicide risk. If a patient is planning to commit suicide, he may give away important belongings (e.g., his favorite piece of clothing) because he believes he will soon be dead and no longer need it. Or a patient may tie up loose ends by calling estranged family members or writing what turn out to be suicide notes to important people in her life. Others may cheek and secretively hoard their pills in preparation for an overdose.

Any major change in the patient's behavior may signal increased risk. For example, patients with personality disorders who have rapid and extreme swings of mood may appear overwhelmed by rage or sadness to the point where they impulsively hurt or kill themselves. As another example, when a sad, withdrawn person suddenly becomes cheerful and energetic, it may be an indication that she has made a detailed suicide plan and is relieved because she feels the end is near. Therefore, the staff should be concerned about patients who change rapidly from deep depression to elation. Similarly, there is reason to doubt the safety of patients who deny suicidal ideation, while at the same time showing behavior that contradicts their denial: making plans to update their will, giving important objects away, or making comments such as "Soon it won't matter any more."

No matter the presentation, one common behavior that increases the risk of suicide is substance abuse. Although alcohol and drugs are prohibited on inpatient psychiatric units, it is sometimes possible for a patient to surreptitiously obtain them. If a patient appears intoxicated or unexplainably sedated, the nurse should consider the possibility of alcohol or drug use. The disinhibiting effects of alcohol or other drugs are often considered to be a final factor that allows someone to make an attempt to end his or her life (Sharfstein, Dickerson, & Oldham, 2009).

Attempts. When patients die by suicide in the hospital, the most common method is by hanging. Patients fashion nooses from available materials, including dental floss, strips of fabric ripped from sheets, or pieces of clothing. The locations of these completed suicides are most often a patient bedroom or bathroom (New York State Office of Mental Health [NYS/OMH], 2009). Other types of attempts made on inpatient units may involve ingestion of drugs or alcohol hidden in patient belongings during admission or brought in by visitors. Similarly, weapons such as razor blades, matches, or knives may be hidden in patient belongings. Occasionally patients will create a weapon from something available on the unit such as a plastic utensil, a pencil, or a broken light bulb.

Cognition

The behaviors of suicidal patients flow directly from their patterns of thinking. Most people with suicidal feelings think pessimistically or negatively about every aspect of their lives. They may ruminate for hours at a time about their perceived failures or about current life crises. They view problems that were normally manageable for them as hopelessly overwhelming and completely insurmountable. Even small tasks like making a bowl of cereal for breakfast or getting out of bed in the morning can be viewed as unmanageable. They have few thoughts of pleasure or hope, even for things that had been enjoyed in the past. Thoughts are end-centered, that is, they focus on failure and death. Even though these thoughts are persistent, there may be moments of ambivalence in which a patient wants to live or doubts her ability to carry out the suicidal plan.

In suicidal patients, thoughts are often experienced as being slowed down or absent, and concentrating becomes difficult. The only topic about which there are detailed thoughts may be suicide, details of the suicide, thoughts about the funeral, thoughts about how individual people in their lives will respond to their death with grief or contrition.

If a patient is psychotic, there may be command hallucinations urging or commanding the patient to kill himself. There may be delusions that causing one's own death is necessary for the welfare of others. For example, the patient may believe that all the evil in the world would be eradicated if he would kill himself.

Affect

Patients at risk for suicide are usually overwhelmed with affect. The most consistent affect in people at risk for suicide is sadness. People sometimes say they feel too bad for sadness—they describe feeling nothing but searing emotional pain and an utter lack of caring about anyone or anything. The despair is so great they cannot imagine how they will make it through the day. They feel hopeless—as if nothing and no one can help them feel like themselves again. They feel helpless—unable to do anything for themselves that would make their lives better. Guilt is prominent and pervasive. Patients often say the world would be better off without them, as would their partners, children, parents, friends, and coworkers. In extreme cases, they feel they don't deserve to remain alive. They see their lives as a series of failures that are now apparent to everyone, thus causing profound embarrassment, humiliation, and shame. They feel unloved, unlovable, and unable to love.

In many suicidal patients, there are deep feelings of loss. Patients say they do not feel like themselves or do not behave in ways that are characteristic of themselves. They may feel they have lost themselves, their sense of humor, their usual sharpness, or their ability to care. Many people also express the feeling they have lost their spiritual connectedness with life and cannot find meaning in anything.

In a sizeable group of people who are at risk for suicide, the feeling of anxiety is even more powerful than the feeling of sadness. These people describe feeling anxious about nearly everything: whether or not to get out of bed; whether to wash their hair; whether they will lose their job or their partner will leave them; whether their children will be irreparably harmed by their illness; and so on. For some, the anxiety takes the form of panic attacks or obsessive thoughts (Townsend, 2009).

Context

Suicide risk is especially high for people with

- A history of previous suicide attempts;
- A family history of completed suicides; or
- Substance abuse

Other known risk factors include

- Psychiatric illness—especially mood disorders such as depression and bipolar disorder;
- Physical illness—especially severe or chronic illness and chronic physical pain;
- Loss—as with a death or loss of a job, financial security, or a relationship;
- Situational crisis—e.g., impending divorce or loss of child custody;
- Particular cultural and religious beliefs (e.g., the belief in traditional Japanese culture that suicide is a noble resolution to a problem);
- Feelings of hopelessness;
- Impulsive or aggressive tendencies; or
- Easy access to lethal methods

(Townsend, 2009, pp. 265–269)

It is worth noting that these risk factors have been identified in outpatient populations and do not necessarily correspond perfectly with the risk factors for people who are psychiatric inpatients. However, there is no research that indicates the precise risk factors specifically for psychiatric inpatients.

Other circumstances are known to be protective; that is, they reduce the risk of suicide. These are

- Concern about effect on family (or sense of responsibility and commitment to family);
- Ability to reality test; i.e., there is an agreement between the patient's perception of the world and the outside world;
- Children in the home;
- Social and/or family support;
- Cognitive flexibility; i.e., the ability to change one's perspective and behavior as situations and circumstances change;

- Pregnancy;
- Religious beliefs that prohibit suicide;
- Positive therapeutic relationship with counselor/therapist;
- Positive coping skills: the ability to talk over problems with others, seek additional information about the situation, break a problem into manageable bits; draw on past experience, make alternative plans for handling a problematic situation, work off tension through physical exercise, or tolerate frustration;
- A cherished animal; or
- If a psychiatric disorder is present, treatment of that disorder

(Worchel & Gearing, 2010)

Suicide may occur in the context of a variety of psychiatric disorders, including major depression, bipolar disorder, schizoaffective disorder, schizophrenia, substance abuse or dependence, anxiety disorders, eating disorders, and personality disorders. Among nonpsychiatric disorders, debilitating and incurable conditions are known to increase the risk of suicide, including multiple sclerosis, heart disease, stroke, severe physical injury, epilepsy, Parkinson's disease, cancers, and dementia.

It is clear from the literature that suicide attempts are twice as common in women, although completed suicide is more common in men. This is partially because men are more likely to use lethal means of suicide such as firearms or jumping from a high place (Townsend, 2009).

POTENTIAL BARRIERS TO BEING THERAPEUTIC

Difficulty in discussing suicide. Suicide and death are difficult topics for many people to discuss, even for health care professionals. One reason for this discomfort is the widespread myth that asking a person about suicide will increase the chances of him having suicidal ideation or behavior. There is no empirical evidence to support this (Townsend, 2009). If a person is not suicidal, talking about suicide will not make them suicidal. On the other hand, if a person is suicidal, talking about it may be a relief.

Suicide has a negative religious or moral connotation for many people who view suicidality as sinful or weak. If this is a patient's view, he may be unwilling to talk about it unless someone else (the nurse) brings it up and clearly demonstrates both verbally and nonverbally an acceptance of the patient's feelings.

There is another important reason a nurse may shy away from talking to patients about suicide: The nurse, too, may have moral or religious beliefs that suicide or even contemplation of suicide is a sign of weakness or religious transgression. The nurse's personal judgment or disapproval has no place in the care of a patient. Yet, these feelings do emerge at times and must be dealt with if the nurse wants to help the patient. It is wise for the nurse to seek supervision if she feels uncomfortable, notices strong negative thoughts about a patient, or is aware that a patient's behavior transgresses strongly held values, or if others notice that she is not behaving in a nonjudgmental way. These feelings are best shared with more experienced colleagues or one's own supervisor in order to move forward with the patient openly and nonjudgmentally (Kneisl & Riley, 2004).

Other reactions the nurse may have. Nurses often have profound emotional reactions to the suicidal patient. Sometimes nurses' responses to their own feelings push the patient away and other times they draw the nurse into overinvolvement with the patient. The following are examples of some unhelpful responses:

- Providing false reassurance (e.g., "You'll be fine")
- Giving advice (e.g., "Just think positive thoughts and you'll feel better")

- Agreeing to keep secrets (i.e., agreeing to keep information to yourself to encourage a patient to confide in you)

Internal beliefs on the part of the nurse can also be problematic, for example:

- Feeling that the nurse is the only person who truly understands the patient or can save the patient
- Planning/wishing to continue contact with the patient after discharge

These are common responses among novice nurses that need to be identified as problematic and discussed in supervision. Having these beliefs is not harmful in itself, but acting on them may be.

Sometimes, difficult feelings, thoughts, or problematic behaviors arise because of countertransference. Countertransference occurs when a nurse responds to a patient as if that patient were someone from his own past. If someone in the nurse's past (including the nurse) has been deeply despairing or suicidal, or if someone close has died by suicide, the nurse may find the feelings related to his own personal experience, such as pain, anger, or helplessness, may arise in relationship to the suicidal patient. This is another situation where supervision is essential. On the rare occasions when these feelings are extreme and the nurse is unable to separate her own personal past experience from the current care of the suicidal patient, it may be necessary for the nurse to concentrate his work on other patients and allow his colleagues for whom this is not a problem to care for the suicidal patient.

Completed suicide. The nurse may be fearful that an acutely suicidal patient will succeed in ending her life. Death of a patient is not common in inpatient psychiatry, yet it does occur. Particularly for relatively inexperienced staff nurses, the fear that they may not be able to prevent the patient's death or self-harm can be terrifying and can lead to overprotecting the patient instead of encouraging self-reliance.

When there has been self-inflicted injury or death of a patient, the caregivers are likely to experience a wide range of deep feelings—guilt, responsibility, sadness, and anger. Staff should have an opportunity to discuss these feelings as a group and individually in supervision. In this situation, the remaining patients on the unit will also need the opportunity to talk about their feelings about the patient's death, both as a group and individually. These feelings can range widely, and may include anger at the staff for not preventing the suicide. Both staff and patients may need some time before they are able to talk about a patient's suicide. No one should be forced to discuss how she feels until she is ready.

OVERVIEW OF NURSING CARE GOALS

1. Safety
   - Prevent suicide or self-harm
2. Stabilization
   - Decrease related psychiatric symptoms
   - Assist the patient in improving coping skills
   - Help the patient develop a relapse prevention plan
3. Engagement
   - Assist patient with engaging in treatment on the unit

When a patient is suicidal, the goal that eclipses all others is keeping the patient safe. Other goals related to stabilization and engagement are also important, but if a conflict in goals arises, the patient's safety always takes precedence.

SAFETY

● **Subgoal: Prevent Suicide or Self-Harm**

Assessment of Risk for Suicide or Self-Harm

In report. Assessment of suicide risk begins in report. When a patient is described as suicidal or having suicidal ideation, the nurse needs clear communication about what the current level of risk is. We discussed risk and protective factors previously; the nurse will begin assessment of these factors in report. Is there a history of suicidal ideation or behavior? If so, the details of time and method are important in assessing risk. Is the individual currently expressing suicidal ideation? If so, does the patient have a plan? If there is a plan, what method is planned and is there any possibility of access to that method? Has the patient harmed herself during the hospitalization? Have any external factors occurred very recently that may be the trigger for more acute risk, such as a loss, a death, or a situational crisis at home?

Finally, it is important for the nursing and other staff to closely communicate about current precautions, such as an increased level of observation, removal of shoelaces or belt, restriction to the unit, and other safeguards.

One-to-one contact. The patient's appearance can provide a great deal of information. Before speaking to the patient it is important to observe affect, posture, degree of eye contact, grooming, hygiene, and degree of agitation or slowing of movement. Sad, anxious, or agitated affect, poor eye contact or hygiene, and psychomotor agitation may all indicate increased suicide risk. Speaking to a suicidal patient is a high priority at the beginning of a shift. The following questions will help elicit information about the current level of risk:

- How are you feeling today? How is your mood?
- How did you sleep last night?

- How is your appetite?
- Have you had any thoughts about harming yourself today? If not, when was the last time you had those thoughts?
- (If the patient has suicidal ideation) Do you have a specific plan? (The nurse will consider whether it is a potentially lethal plan, as well as whether the patient might access the means to carry out the plan.)
- (If the patient is psychotic) Have you heard any voices telling you to hurt yourself or someone else?
- The nurse will also ask about any other symptoms that have been especially troubling, such as anxiety, fear, or helplessness.

If the patient is expressing suicidal ideation, the nurse can ask the patient to rate the strength of the ideation on a scale of 0 to 10, where 0 is no suicidal ideation and 10 is the strongest suicidal feelings ever felt. This numerical rating will serve as a baseline measure of degree of suicidality against which the nurse can compare either improvement or worsening. However, it is also important to note that suicidal patients may not be completely forthcoming about their thoughts or plans about suicide, and the nurse should look for inconsistencies between a denial of suicidality and actual behaviors.

On the unit. The nurse's observations of the patient on the unit provide further information about risk factors. Behaviors that may indicate a higher suicidal risk include isolation, refusal of meals, crying, inability to sleep, expressions of hopelessness or suicidal intent, inquiries about methods of suicide, agitation, impulsivity, or refusal to talk about the future.

Supportive visits and phone calls may serve as factors protecting the patient from self-harm or suicide. Having a positive relationship with a staff member or another patient may also be protective. Lack of protective factors place patients at higher risk.

● Key Nursing Interventions to Prevent Suicide or Self-Harm

Maintain a safe environment. Inpatient psychiatric units are designed to provide a safe environment. There should be no sharp objects or potential weapons available to patients. The furniture and hardware on the entire unit should be designed to minimize the risk for self-injury. A careful search of the patient's belongings before arrival on the inpatient unit should assure that no dangerous objects remain.

Even though environmental dangers have been minimized, a patient with intense suicidal ideation may find a way to hurt or kill himself using objects or substances on the unit or brought in by visitors. Therefore, when a patient is suicidal, the nurse's observations of the safety of the unit are paramount. On regular rounds or checks of the unit, nurses need to be alert to any environmental risks such as unattended keys or an unlocked treatment room door. When visitors arrive or other patients return from pass, the nurse must be diligent to check all items brought in from outside the hospital lest a dangerous item be brought in and made available.

Because most suicide attempt in hospitals occur by hanging in either a bathroom or bedroom, these are areas of special importance. Ideally, a suicidal patient should be assigned a room in close proximity to the nurses' station. For patients who can tolerate a roommate during this critical stage, they may find a roommate to be an additional short-term source of support or comfort. If the hospital has rooms with specially designed safe hardware, the suicidal patient should occupy one of these rooms. There may be instances in which the nurses need to remove furniture that is questionable from the patient's room. The nurse may need to carefully evaluate the safety of objects ordinarily supplied to patients, such as razors for shaving or shoes with shoelaces. If the nurse determines these items are unsafe, it is important to let family and friends know they cannot bring these items to the hospital for the patient until the patient recovers. Sometimes, another patient will confide in the staff that a suicidal patient has a razor blade or pills or some other instrument of self-harm. If there is any question about the patient having a dangerous object or substance, extensive room and body searches must be conducted according to hospital policy. Because body searches are intrusive, they should not be carried out unless there is substantial reason to believe the patient may be hiding a dangerous object on his person. When body searches are done, the nurse will follow appropriate hospital policies, which likely include the following: The nurse should ensure that the person doing the search is the same sex as the patient, has appropriate training in doing this type of search, and that there is another same-sex staff member in the room. Body searches should include careful attention to the hair, hems of clothing, and patient's shoes, where dangerous objects or substances may be secreted.

Increase direct patient contact. Level of observation is obviously an important decision with the suicidal patient. Although this ultimately is the decision of the physician, nurses have a great deal of input into that decision based on assessment of key risk and protective factors, acute behavior changes, and observations of the patient's behavior. It is important for the nurse to communicate with the team when she or he has observed something that may indicate increased risk of imminent suicidal behavior.

When restrictions are placed on the patient, for example, restriction to the unit or one-to-one observation, the nurse needs to clearly tell the patient exactly what the restrictions will be and that their purpose will be to keep the patient safe. For example, when telling the patient that she will be on one-to-one observation, the nurse needs to let her know that this observation will continue at all times, including during sleep and when using the bathroom or shower. The nurse should communicate that all restrictions are being put in place to keep the patient safe, and that the restrictions will continue only until the extreme suicidal urges abate.

If a patient is on one-to-one observation, the staff member must find a way to maintain direct visual observation at all times, even when the patient is showering or using the bathroom. No activity can be allowed that would distract the staff member from constant, undivided attention to the safety of the patient. Because this level of observation is intrusive to the patient and absorbs all the attention of one staff member at the expense of the other patients, it should be reserved only for patients at extreme risk for suicide or self-harm.

The nurse can give feedback to the team regarding reductions in acute suicide risk (reduced risk factors, increased protective factors) and the patient may be changed to a less restrictive level of observation according to hospital policy.

Provide education to the patient and explore ambivalence. The nurse may hear many statements of hopelessness and discouragement. It is important that the nurse view these as true reflections of the patient's internal feeling state without either accepting them as "objective truth" or attempting to stop the patient from expressing or feeling them. As part of educating the patient about suicidal feelings, the nurse could counsel the patient that the current feelings, though very intense and real at this moment, may change over time. In other words, it may be wise to let the patient know that they may see their current problems differently or more positively when the suicidal crisis passes. For example, the nurse may say, "I can't even imagine how terrible you must feel right now, but I want you to know that many people respond to treatment and feel better over time."

If the patient expresses ambivalence about suicide, the nurse should encourage the patient to explore the side of the ambivalence that protects him from making an attempt—in other words, the factors that make the patient want to live. If the patient expresses no ambivalence, it may be helpful to ask the patient if he experiences any misgivings or ambivalence about dying. By encouraging the patient to explore his own wish to live, even though it may be a very small part of his current emotional state, the nurse may help the patient balance out his self-destructive feelings. When the patient is not in touch with any reason to live or feel hope, the nurse can let the patient know that the staff will care for him until he can care for himself again.

Do not rely on no-harm contracts. An agreement or no-harm contract can be discussed with the patient; however, it is unsafe to rely on a no-harm contract as the only or the primary intervention (Lynch, Howard, El-Mallakh, & Matthews, 2008). If used, this type of agreement MUST always be only a part of a comprehensive treatment plan.

Ensure clear staff communication. Because safety is a life or death issue for these patients, teamwork and communication are especially important. All disciplines must plan and work together, as must staff on all shifts. Every team member must know which precautions to take with a suicidal patient and carry them out consistently. If there are times of day or particular situations that exacerbate the patient's suicidality, everyone caring for the patient needs to know about them. If one staff member becomes aware of the appearance of a new risk factor for suicide, it must be communicated quickly to other members of the team. If different members of the team disagree about the best approach to a suicidal patient, having an open discussion about the plan of care can help clarify the best course of action.

STABILIZATION

● Subgoal: Decrease Related Psychiatric Symptoms

Assessment of Related Psychiatric Symptoms

In report. Because suicidal patients have so many different presentations and associated symptoms, it is important to select a few key target symptoms for each individual that seem to be most distressing and are potentially related to suicidality. Target symptoms will be selected in collaboration with the patient and discussed in report. Sample target symptoms include hopelessness, insomnia, isolation, agitation, refusing medications, command hallucinations, and poor grooming and hygiene. For each target symptom, it is important to define the symptom in a measurable way so that all staff can communicate effectively on its occurrence. For example, if insomnia is a symptom, how many actual hours of sleep did the patient get? If appetite is a target, what percent of each meal was consumed?

By using target symptoms with clearly defined measurements, staff can report the patient's progress in a way that can be understood by all. In report, the nurse needs to learn the status of all the patient's target symptoms.

One-to-one contact. The one-to-one encounter is a chance to select target symptoms and verify the status of the target symptoms given in report. If the nurse and patient agree on target symptoms, then both can observe for improvement in an objective way. The nurse should ask questions such as "Overall, how are you feeling about your progress?" "What has been most helpful?" "Is there anything the staff can provide to help you in recovery?"

On the unit. Observing the patient in everyday activities can help the nurse gauge his progress on target symptoms. As the patient stabilizes, the nurse may notice an improvement in posture, grooming, hygiene, sleep, appetite, and engagement with others. The patient's movements may become more animated, and she may begin to show some feelings other than sadness or despair. This gradual improvement differs from a more sudden and dramatic improvement in mood that may indicate relief at having decided on a definite suicide plan. The nurse should continue to track the patient's target symptoms throughout the day.

● **Key Nursing Interventions to Reduce Related Psychiatric Symptoms**

Provide access to peer support and other resources to decrease hopelessness. For many suicidal individuals, hopelessness and/or isolation are key related symptoms; peer support can help to alleviate these symptoms. Suicidal individuals may feel hopeless to tolerate the extreme feelings they experience or hopeless that they will ever feel well again or feel like themselves again. As they stabilize, it is often helpful to introduce them to others who have recovered more fully and may be able to provide hope and insight. Some hospitals employ peer advocates who can visit patients and share their stories of recovery. Other hospitals have on-site meetings of support groups such as the National Alliance on Mental Illness or the Depressive and Bipolar Support Alliance. If patients have access to the Internet, they can visit the websites of these organizations. It is common for hospitals to provide patients with written or audiovisual information about their symptoms or illness, which can have a similar effect of providing hope. Early in the stabilization period, these materials will be most helpful if they are brief and simple. As the patient's ability to think and concentrate improves, she may be interested in more in-depth information. The patient may also continue to use these resources after the hospitalization.

Address hopelessness and depression directly. When patients are suicidal in the context of a depression, they often blame themselves (Joiner Jr, Van Orden, Witte, & Rudd, 2009). In these cases, it is important to teach that "depression is an illness and not a weakness." The hopelessness and guilt that patients experience are cardinal symptoms of depression. That is, they are a part of the illness; they are symptoms that can change with time. When these patients recover, they may be able to see the identical life situation differently. What now seems overwhelming and hopeless may seem easier to manage once their mood has returned to normal. While patients may not seem to believe this information at the time, there may be a small part of them that hears the nurse say this, and hopes it will be true.

Provide medications appropriate for target symptoms. Benzodiazepines may be prescribed to reduce anxiety during the day or to improve sleep at night. Other non-benzodiazepine sedatives, sedating antidepressants, or sedating antihistamines may also be ordered to improve sleep. Antidepressants or mood stabilizers may be prescribed for depressive symptoms and antipsychotics for psychotic symptoms. The patient will need to know which of these medications are to be used as needed for symptom relief and which should be taken regularly as standing doses.

● **Subgoal: Assist the Patient in Improving Coping Skills**

Assessment of Coping Skills

In report. In report, it is important to hear about the patient's use of coping skills. If he is learning dialectical behavioral therapy or cognitive behavioral therapy skills, has he been using them? Has he found successful ways to self-soothe? Has he practiced any of the relaxation skills he is learning or used any personal stress-reducing methods such as listening to music, journaling, or practicing abdominal breathing? If so, how successful were these methods?

One-to-one contact. Suicidal patients may have a paucity of coping methods. The nurse can help them learn new ways to reduce stress and symptoms, ways to self-soothe when suicidal thinking begins to form, and ways to increase support during symptomatic periods. As with all people, what is helpful to one patient may not be to another. Patients must discover ways to cope that work for them as individuals.

The nurse can begin this process by asking the patient what works for her to reduce stress and symptoms, self-soothe, and increase support. The patient may have difficulty naming an activity that she can engage in to meet these criteria, so it may help to ask what she enjoyed doing in the past before she was ill.

On the unit. Observing the patient's ordinary activities and interactions allows the nurse to determine what coping skills the patient relies on and how effective they are. As the patient learns new coping skills, the nurse will watch to see if they are being used in day-to-day interaction and activities on the unit.

● **Key Nursing Interventions to Increase Coping Skills**

Help patients to identify and use useful coping methods. Teaching about stress management and coping skills can be a pleasant experience for the nurse and patient. A good place to begin is to discuss the patient's current and past strategies for coping with stress and to attempt to understand which have been most effective in the past and could be used going forward. Coping methods that are harmful or not effective, such as self-injury or drug use, cannot be eliminated unless there are alternative methods available.

Once the nurse has assessed the patient's current and past coping skills, the nurse can offer other, alternative methods to add to the patient's repertory, asking the patient to choose the ones that appeal to him. To some degree, the options offered will depend upon the philosophy and therapeutic approach of the unit. In all cases, some of the suggestions may include the following: use of whatever has worked in the past, such as fishing, yoga, walking outdoors, and curling up with a favorite pet; use of sensory modalities, such as aromatherapy, massage, drinking herbal tea, and taking a hot bath; journaling or completing crossword puzzles; exercise; relaxation exercises such as deep breathing or progressive muscle relaxation; dancing; or listening to music (Townsend, 2009). Reaching out to a specific person might also be important.

In terms of stress management, one of the most important measures is structuring one's time by planning ahead to keep oneself occupied in fulfilling and meaningful activities, punctuated by periods of relaxation and leisure. This work can begin in the hospital by helping the patient create a healthy and balanced schedule on the unit.

Patients often underestimate the importance of healthy eating, adequate sleep, and regular exercise in furthering their recovery. Teaching patients about these three aspects of overall health is one of the most important lessons the nurse can impart to help them get well and stay well.

● Subgoal: Help the Patient Develop a Relapse Prevention Plan

A relapse prevention plan includes a list of warning signs (i.e., key symptoms) that often precede the onset of suicidal ideation or behavior, a list of situational or behavioral triggers that may lead to these warning signs, and a plan for coping with each of the specific symptoms or triggers. It may also include a plan for living an overall healthy lifestyle.

Assess When Patient Is Ready for Relapse Prevention

In report. A nurse may hear in report that a patient who is beginning to stabilize is asking how to prevent future episodes of suicidal ideation or behavior, or worrying about her ability to prevent them. This signals that the patient is ready to begin planning for relapse prevention.

One-to-one contact. It is sometimes difficult for a suicidal patient in recovery to entertain the thought that relapse is possible. By expressing every hope that the symptoms of suicidality will never return, the nurse can reassure the patient that although relapse is possible, it can be prevented or the severity lessened if the early warning signs are identified and managed immediately. Having a relapse prevention plan in place is like having insurance against relapse.

The one-to-one contact is a good time to assess whether the patient is ready to learn more about their illness and treatment, including their medication(s). This is the first step to developing a relapse prevention plan. The nurse might begin by asking if the patient feels ready to talk more about illness and recovery. Does the patient know which medications she is taking and how that medication is expected to help? Does she understand the circumstances or factors that led to her suicidal feelings? Would she like to learn more?

On the unit. Increased engagement in unit activities may signal that the patient is ready to work on relapse prevention.

● **Key Nursing Interventions to Assist Patient With Developing a Relapse Prevention Plan**

Help the patient to understand the course and pattern of symptoms. As a patient becomes less overtly suicidal, the nurse can help the patient educate himself about the course and pattern of their symptoms, with a particular focus on the suicidality. When did suicidal thoughts or behaviors begin? What was happening in the patient's life at the time the symptoms first appeared? Have the symptoms been constant, or have they arisen in response to particular stresses or circumstances? What has made the symptoms milder? What has made them more severe? Is this problem one that the patient shares with other members of her family? Does she think this is a pattern developed independently, or might it be part of a genetic or familial pattern, either inherited or learned? This may lead to an understanding of warning signs of suicidality, as well as understanding that the patient does not *always* feel suicidal. Finally, this may give the patient some distance from the suicidal thoughts so that the patient can realize she does not always have to act on her thoughts.

Help the patient identify warning signs that suicidal feelings are in danger of returning. Warning signs are symptoms that often precede suicidality. By carefully reviewing the symptoms that preceded the current and past episodes of suicidality, the patient can create a personalized list. These warning signs will differ from patient to patient and may include loss of appetite, lack of interest in things previously enjoyed, trouble concentrating, isolating oneself, being overly sensitive to sound or light, sleeping excessively, and being irritable.

Help the patient to identify triggers of suicidality. The next step is to help the patient identify triggers, which are situations or actions that triggered the warning signs in the past. Triggers, like warning signs, are quite individual. For some, the most reliable trigger will be losing a night's sleep due to external circumstances such as travel or a family emergency. For others, it may be spending a certain holiday with family; alcohol or other drug use; spending time with negative people; or taking on too much responsibility. Avoiding these triggers is one of the most powerful things a patient can do to prevent relapse, but it may be difficult. For example, if spending a holiday with family is a trigger, how can the patient avoid being with family for the holiday without hurting them unduly? If drug or alcohol use is a trigger, what are specific ways the patient can avoid temptation to use? Helping the patient think through specific ways to avoid their own personal triggers—and writing them down for future reference—can be very helpful.

Assist the patient with making a relapse prevention plan. A relapse prevention plan is easiest to follow when it is created by or with the patient and written down so it can be referred to regularly. A complete plan consists of a list of environmental triggers of suicidal ideation and behavior and specific ways to avoid them. Personal warning signs (or symptoms) that typically precede suicide ideation or behavior should also be listed and matched up with specific measures to be taken in the event that symptoms occur. This, too, is specific to the individual and can be identified by asking the patient to think about things he can do to help himself feel better when he is feeling stressed or out of sorts. This list often includes contacting specific support persons; reducing personal stress; setting aside time for relaxation, rest, or enjoyment; and use of other specific coping strategies. The more concrete the list, the better.

An overall health-promoting lifestyle may be a part of the plan. The nurse can ask the patient what she needs to do every day in order to feel well. Creating a plan to include these activities on a daily basis can empower the patient to be in charge of her own health.

Teach about expected course of illness. Everyone, even people who are recovering from a suicidal crisis, has better and worse days. Patients and their friends and family members need to know that recovery is not always linear, and there will be peaks and valleys. It may be helpful for the nurse to tell the patient what feelings, thoughts, or behaviors can usually be expected in a normal recovery from a suicidal crisis. This can help the patient to de-catastrophize and seek help when he has a bad day.

TREATMENT ENGAGEMENT

● **Subgoal: Assist Patient With Engaging in Treatment on the Unit**

Assessment of Ability to Engage in Treatment on the Unit

As the suicidal patient stabilizes, the nurse's ability to engage her in treatment to the fullest extent possible is greatly enhanced. While the patient is still in a suicidal crisis, it is difficult, if not impossible, to reach out to anyone, particularly in the first hours and days when the nurse and the patient are strangers to one another. As the patient's symptoms abate, establishing a relationship becomes a possibility, keeping in mind the relationship is built on trust.

There are many early signs of engagement: when a patient begins to talk about symptoms with the staff, when the patient accepts medication for the first time, or when the patient first asks the nurse for help of even the most minor sort. Simply being able to admit having suicidal feelings or urges is a major step for some patients. If those early attempts at connection are successful, the way is paved for fuller engagement. Gradually, the patient should begin to interact with different staff members and patients. Participating in groups on the unit and asking questions about the treatment plan are also good signs of progression. Ultimately, full engagement occurs when the patient takes primary responsibility for recovery from the suicidal crisis, so any attempt on the patient's part to better understand the events and circumstances that led to suicidality indicates movement in that direction. Similarly, efforts to understand the details of treatment, recovery, and self-management indicate that the patient is becoming an active participant. The nurse should see a progression in engagement on good days, and more importantly, should see that the patient can connect with the nurse on the patient's bad days when some degree of suicidal thinking or despair may reoccur.

One barrier to engagement is the experience of increasing symptoms after a period of improvement. The nurse should watch for this. Because it is often difficult for patients to ask for help when they are experiencing a return of symptoms, it is useful to have collateral sources of information beyond what the nurse hears in report and sees on the unit. It is not uncommon for information about a turn for the worse in a suicidal patient to come from a source other than the patient. It may be that another patient is worried about an interaction with the suicidal patient and shares that worry with staff, or a friend or family member had an alarming phone conversation with the patient and contacts a staff member. The nurse should use these reports as an opportunity to approach the patient and attempt to engage him in the treatment process once again.

● **Key Nursing Interventions to Increase Engagement in Treatment**

Assist patient with understanding seriousness of his situation. Some patients deny that suicidality is a real issue for them, as minimizing the event makes it easier to bear. They may believe it was a momentary response to a stressor in their lives that is unlikely to ever recur. Or they may tell the nurse they were just kidding when they said they were suicidal and that people are taking them too seriously. These reports may not match with the apparent seriousness of the crisis (e.g., the patient had clearly made preparations to kill herself). For some patients, the most effective way to help them come to terms with the seriousness of their situation is to provide them with articles, DVDs, or books that tell the stories of other people who have survived a suicidal crisis (Townsend, 2009). When helping patients to understand the seriousness of suicidality, it is important to balance this with hope for a better future.

Increase the likelihood that the patient can confide his symptoms. While talking with a suicidal person, it is important to help the patient feel safe and free to talk. It is often difficult for these patients to discuss their feelings. In fact, it is sometimes difficult for suicidal patients to talk at all. Their speech may be spare and halting, in which case, it is important to allow them time to express themselves. Often they are in a frame of mind to harshly judge themselves, so it is important for them to perceive no judgment from the nurse. Remaining calm, unhurried, and relaxed may help this patient to open up (Townsend, 2009). Cultural, family, or religious values may make this especially challenging for some. When a patient denies suicidal ideation but exhibits behaviors that indicate the opposite, for example, sudden and complete withdrawal from peers, it may help to point out the discrepancy between their actions and their words in a gentle fashion. In all cases, a nonjudgmental and supportive approach on the part of the nurse is essential. If a nurse becomes aware that an individual is hesitant to admit suicidal feelings, it may help to discuss with that individual the importance of sharing symptoms and the risks of holding back. That is, when the patient shares her symptoms with a nurse, the nurse can be in a position to help in some way. In the hospital, the suicidal patient is always asked to inform a staff member if she is having suicidal thoughts.

Attempt to increase willingness to take medications. Patients for whom medications are a part of treatment should be educated about every aspect of their medications: names, doses, schedule, mechanism of action, side effects, and course of treatment. Patients can be empowered to be partners in treatment, providing real-time feedback about ways in which the medication is helping or causing discomfort.

Because many psychotropic medications do not work right away, patients usually suffer from side effects while still in the hospital and before the medication has had a chance to start reducing their symptoms. Under these circumstances, the patient will feel worse than he did before he started taking the medication. This can strain the patient's relationship with treatment staff, may decrease treatment engagement, and may increase the risk that the patient will stop taking the medication. The good news is that most side effects will disappear on their own in a few days or weeks if the patient can tolerate them for that length of time. This is important to convey to the patient along with a great deal of reassurance and any conservative measures that will make the side effects more tolerable until they abate. For example, a headache may respond to acetaminophen, and complaints of sedation may be more tolerable with a few brief rest periods throughout the day. By ensuring that medication side effects are as mild as possible and that the patient understands them, the nurse can strengthen the patient's engagement in treatment.

One of the problems for patients with chronic mental illness, particularly those with a history of suicidality, is the double-edged sword of good medication response. On the one hand, most psychotropics help ameliorate symptoms. In many cases, they return the patient to a life much like that before the problems began. On the other hand, a patient may do such a good job that after 6 months or a year or 10 years, the patient may begin to doubt she needs to continue taking medication. Regardless of how long a patient has been stable, for patients with chronic illness, stopping the medication will increase the risk of relapse. The nurse needs to educate the patient and family that stopping or reducing the dose of a medication without collaboration with the health care provider may lead to relapse and a return of suicidal thoughts or behaviors.

PREPARATION FOR DISCHARGE

Plan for a safe home environment. As the patient recovers, the entire treatment team will need to think about the safety of their home environment as well, especially in regard to any potential weapons or other available means of suicide. If a patient hoarded pills for an overdose before admission, a friend or family member can dispose of those pills. Any potential weapons will need to be secured or removed from the home. Access to weapons in the homes of family and friends also needs to be addressed—family and friends who may have weapons need to secure them as well.

Planning for a suicidal crisis. In the event of a suicidal crisis, patients need to know how to contact their local emergency room or crisis team after discharge. These phone numbers, along with the numbers for 24-hour crisis and suicide hotlines, should be written down for the patient and kept in a safe and accessible place. This can be presented to the patient as the final coping skill if none of the others in the relapse prevention plan are providing adequate relief (Kneisl & Riley, 2004).

TABLE 9.1
Goals, Areas of Assessment, and Interventions for a
Patient With Suicide

Goal	Assessment	Intervention
Safety		
Prevent suicide or self-harm	Assess risk and protective factors and current suicidal ideation and behavior, using information from all sources including direct patient inquiry Assess environmental safety	Maintain a safe environment Increase direct patient contact Provide education to the patient and explore ambivalence Do not rely on no-harm contracts Ensure clear staff communication
Stabilization		
Decrease related psychiatric symptoms	Select and assess key target symptoms that are related to suicidality. Sample target symptoms include: hopelessness, insomnia, isolation, agitation, refusing medications, command hallucinations, and poor grooming and hygiene Track status of target symptoms	Provide access to peer support and other resources to decrease hopelessness Address depression and hopelessness directly Provide medications appropriate for target symptoms
Assist the patient in improving coping skills	Know coping skills that the patient is currently learning Ask patient about coping skills that have been helpful in the past Assess use of newly introduced coping skills	Help patients to identify and use useful coping methods

(cont.)

TABLE 9.1
Goals, Areas of Assessment, and Interventions for a
Patient With Suicide *(cont.)*

Goal	Assessment	Intervention
Stabilization		
Help the patient develop a relapse prevention plan	Determine readiness to discuss relapse prevention Assess whether the patient is ready to learn more about their illness and its treatment	Help the patient to understand course and pattern of symptoms Help the patient to identify warning signs Help the patient to identify triggers of suicidality Assist the patient with making a relapse prevention plan Teach about expected course of illness
Treatment Engagement		
Assist patient with engaging in treatment on the unit	Watch for early signs of engagement such as talking with staff about symptoms, accepting medications, or asking for help Observe whether patient is participating in groups on the unit Assess interest in understanding illness and treatment Watch for barriers to engagement, such as return of symptoms	Assist patient with understanding the seriousness of her situation Increase the likelihood that the patient can confide his symptoms Attempt to increase willingness to take medications

REFERENCES

Joiner, T. E., Jr., VanOrden, K. A., Witte, T. K., & Rudd, M. D. (2009). Guidance for working with suicidal clients. In *The interpersonal theory of suicide* (pp. 26–27). Washington, DC: American Psychological Association.

Kneisl, C. R., & Riley, E. A. (2004). Clients at risk for suicide and self-destructive behavior. In C. R. Kneisel, H. S. Wilson, & E. Trigoboff (Eds.), *Contemporary psychiatric-mental health nursing* (pp. 526–542). Upper Saddle River, NJ: Pearson Prentice Hall.

Lynch, M. A., Howard, P. B., El-Mallakh, P., & Matthews, J. M. (2008). Assessment and management of hospitalized suicidal patients. *Journal of Psychosocial Nursing and Mental Health Services, 46,* 45–52.

Munich, R. L., & Greene, P. K. (2009). Psychosocial approaches in inpatient psychiatry. In F. Ovsiew, & R. L. Munich (Eds.), *Principles of inpatient psychiatry* (pp. 17–41). Philadelphia, PA: Lippincott Williams & Wilkins.

New York State Office of Mental Health. (2009). *Incident Reports and Root Cause Analyses 2002–2008: What They Reveal About Suicides.* Retrieved March 10, 2011, from http://www.omh.ny.gov/omhweb/statistics/suicide_incident_rpt/

Sharfstein, S. S., Dickerson, F. B., & Oldham, J. M. (2009). *Textbook of hospital psychiatry.* Arlington, VA: American Psychiatric Publishing.

Townsend, M. C. (2009). The suicidal client. In E. M. Varcarolis & M. J. Halter (Ed.), *Psychiatric mental health nursing* (pp. 264–278). Philadelphia, PA: FA Davis.

Worchel, D., & Gearing, R. E. (2010). *Suicide assessment and treatment empirical and evidence based practices.* New York: Springer Publishing.

The Patient Who Is Withdrawn

10

Mary Leveillee, Christopher Towey,
Emily McCue, Kevin Ritchie,
Judy L. Sheehan, Joanne M. Matthew,
and Lisa A. Uebelacker

BACKGROUND AND DESCRIPTION

In this chapter, we discuss two kinds of withdrawal: passive withdrawal and active withdrawal. Passive withdrawal refers to when patients appear to lack energy and motivation required for engagement. Active withdrawal appears as a more a deliberate act of holding back from engagement or refusing treatment and can range from partial or selective to complete withdrawal. Active withdrawal is a more energized withdrawal, and the patient may seem agitated, anxious, angry, or frustrated (for some of these patients, Chapter 1, "The Patient With Anger," or Chapter 2, "The Patient With Anxiety," may be useful.) Patients can vacillate between passive and active withdrawal.

Behavior

A patient who is passively withdrawn may appear inhibited, muted, isolated, and with restricted affect. This patient may seem lethargic or apathetic and may have difficulty engaging in one-to-one interactions and tolerating group activity. He avoids the milieu, staying in his room, or if out on the unit, sitting alone, sometimes with closed eyes. If the withdrawal is based on fear, staff may note that the patient scans the environment or sits in a place where he can see the rest of the unit. The patient who is passively withdrawn may not be eating regularly because of an intolerance of the milieu.

Catatonia is a form of passive withdrawal. Catatonia can involve either severe psychomotor retardation or agitation. The patient who is catatonic may seem like a statue, maintaining the same posture for hours. He will stare without blinking and will often not swallow spontaneously, which leads to drooling. In this inhibited state, the patient may also be mute. Conversely, catatonia can also appear as agitated, repetitive, purposeless motion. The patient may exhibit echolalia and echopraxia, that is, the repeating of words and motions of others. It is possible that if the nurse actively repositions the patient, such as when taking vital signs, the patient's arm will stay in the air as if the nurse is still taking her pulse. This ability to "pose" the patient is called waxy flexibility. In both the active and the inhibited presentation, the patient with catatonia can have a resistance to all attempts to move her ignoring requests or commands (i.e., negativism) and not responding to verbal or physical prompts (Penland, Weder & Tampi, 2006, pp. 2–3). At times, the nurse may foster a change in posture with directive verbal commands: "Anne, please walk to the bathroom with me."

Patients demonstrating active withdrawal may demonstrate refusal to engage in treatment interventions. This is the patient who will not allow his vital signs to be taken, who refuses medical interventions such as monitoring of blood sugar, or who refuses to take some or all medications. There are times when active withdrawal may include behaviors that create physical vulnerability such as refusal to eat or engage in activities of daily living. Many times active withdrawal involves preoccupation with one's own physical well-being as seen in somatization disorders, and engagement with others will be limited to voicing and attending to those fears. Actively withdrawn patients may request to leave against medical advice, citing that treatment is ineffective or that they are no longer in need of treatment. These patients may also make threatening statements such as "You better leave me alone if you know what is good for you" or "Tell them to stay out of my face."

There are times when a patient may demonstrate selective active withdrawal by refusing only certain elements of treatment. The patient may take medications but will not engage in the milieu or one-to-one interactions, or she may talk only with certain staff and be selective in the groups she will attend.

Cognition

Passive withdrawal may be associated with many types of thought processes. Those who are depressed may be experiencing increased confusion, difficulty with fluidly connecting thoughts in conversation, poor sense of self-worth, hopelessness, guilt, or ruminative thought process. A ruminative thought process is one that is highly focused on one or two ideas that often relate to despondent themes such as loss, despair, guilt, or hopelessness. The person may become lost in thoughts of "if only I had..." or "my life is over because..." or even be replaying painful events repeatedly. The person can become so absorbed in these thoughts that she is unable to engage in present-focused discussion and problem solving.

The patient who is withdrawn may also experience obsessive thoughts and as a result of phobias or obsessions have a fear of interaction. Patients with dementia may appear withdrawn due to confusion and an inability to process the environment. The patient who is paranoid may experience thoughts that people in the milieu are there to hurt her or spy on her and withdraw as a result. Patients may have auditory hallucinations that involve voices telling them that others are dangerous or they need to stay away from others.

Active withdrawal or refusal of treatment similarly may be associated with a variety of cognitive processes. In these patients, thoughts might include "no one here can help me," "no one actually cares," "they don't get me," or "they are all out to get me." Refusal of treatment could be due to fears of contamination (i.e., as seen in obsessive–compulsive disorder) or paranoia about being poisoned. Active withdrawal may occur because a patient is confused (perhaps due to dementia or delirium) and/or is attempting to control her environment in any way possible. Finally, active withdrawal may be due to a previous negative experience with hospitalization or treatment.

Affect

Many different emotions may underlie withdrawn behavior. First, fear is very common. Fear is clearly evident in the patient who is paranoid or anxious or has dementia. Their fears and feelings of vulnerability may lead them to withdraw as a form of self-protection. Some patients may present as irritable or angry but fear may be underlying the anger. Other patients may be fearful of the environment or other people because of hallucinations. At times, the voices can also be threatening; this amplifies the fear a patient will experience.

Second, some patients may experience sadness, hopelessness, apathy, a feeling of emptiness, a diminishment of feeling, or a lack of interest and motivation.

Third, shame can underlie withdrawn behavior. Shame is an undercurrent in many patients with histories of abuse, and coupled with the anxiety seen in posttraumatic stress, it can inhibit their ability to communicate about their internal struggle to treatment providers. Self-injurious behaviors often lead to shame and embarrassment as the patient may feel embarrassed about discussing her self-injury. The patient may choose not to engage in treatment so as to minimize or avoid feelings of shame.

Finally, anger may be associated with withdrawn behaviors. As mentioned above, some patients may act out in angry ways as an expression of their fear and desire to keep others at a distance. Some patients experience anger when they do not believe they have a problem but come into the hospital due to pressure from family or for safety reasons. These patients may reject whatever aspects of treatment are in their power to reject. Other patients are in the hospital voluntarily but experience discomfort and blame the staff for not being efficient or caring enough to ease their process. Finally, some patients may want to engage in treatment but be unable to for some reason; these patients may show frustration related to inability to express themselves or be understood in a satisfactory manner.

Context

Active and passive withdrawal can be seen across the spectrum of psychiatric disorders, including anxiety disorders, mood disorders, substance abuse, eating disorders, personality disorders, and psychotic disorders, as well as in patients with dementia or delirium. Those that are depressed will demonstrate withdrawal because of slowed cognitive processes and psychomotor retardation. In schizophrenia, apathy is a part of the negative signs and symptoms. Catatonia may also be seen in other psychiatric conditions such as depressive disorders, bipolar disorder, schizophrenia, and dementia (Penland et al., 2006).

There are other reasons for withdrawal. Hospitalization is stressful, and some patients may withdraw in order to cope with stress of illness or hospitalization (DeNuccio & Schwartz-Barcott, 2000). Other possible sources of withdrawal behavior include barriers to communication such as cultural or language barriers. Physical limitations such as hearing impairment, arthritis or fibromyalgia pain, or other physical problems that result in being easily fatigued may limit the time a patient can sit and interact. (Fortinash & Holoday-Worret, 2008; Townsend, 2008; Vacarolis & Halter, 2010; Videbeck, 2011.)

POTENTIAL BARRIERS TO BEING THERAPEUTIC

It is very easy to become frustrated and angry with the patient who is not responding to efforts of support and help, and the nurse can feel as if this is a personal rejection or a negative statement about his skill in care delivery. This is particularly true when a patient seems to respond selectively to some staff but not others. As summarized by Breeze and Repper (1998), "threats to the nurses' competence and control are important factors when defining patients as 'difficult'" (p. 1303). For the withdrawn patient, the nurse can also become frustrated due to the repetitive nature of both interventions and the patient's responses. Alternatively or in addition, nurses may have a response of sadness or hopelessness.

OVERVIEW OF NURSING CARE GOALS

1. Safety
   - Prevent passive self-harm
   - Prevent harm to others
2. Stabilization and engagement
   - Help patient to decrease withdrawal and increase treatment engagement

---

Note that we consider stabilization and engagement together when addressing withdrawn behavior as engagement represents stabilization for these patients.

SAFETY

● **Subgoal: Prevent Passive Self-Harm**

Assessment of Risk for Passive Self-Harm

Passive self-harm refers to problems such as poor nutrition, poor hydration, lack of self-care, and refusal of necessary medications. Inhibited mobility as seen in catatonia or severe psychomotor retardation makes self-care impossible, and it is necessary that the nurse takes an active role in intervention. Patients with catatonia are at risk for severe complications, including malnutrition, dehydration, contractures, and pulmonary emboli (Penland, et al., 2006, p. 4).

In report. Immediate risk assessment involves discussion of the patient's well being and communication of vital signs, sleeping and eating patterns, hydration, respiration, speech, sensorium, and gait as objective measures of physical well being. If the patient is refusing nursing assessment and interventions, then observational measures become essential in staff communication and decision making. Nurses must also be aware of the patient's medical history in order to understand the particular risks to the patient who is inactive, not eating, or not adhering to medical treatments. Nurses should report on any active assessments or interventions that were needed in the previous shift (e.g., checking skin integrity or bathing the patient).

One-to-one contact. As the nurse is able to engage the patient, he should explore concerns related to passive self-harm by asking questions such as, "I noticed you really didn't eat. How is your appetite?" or "You didn't seem to like the dinner, is there anything else I can get you?" Starting with a global exploration of the patient's experience is less threatening than asking "why" questions regarding her refusal of care.

As the conversation continues, the nurse will gently explore the patient's underlying thought process to understand why he may be refusing food, water, or medications. Patients may simply have their own routines with food intake and self-care, so exploring "how you usually do things" will help shed light on how the unit routine may be disruptive and provide avenues of mutual agreement. For example, the nurse may say, "Tell me what a normal day of eating is like for you when you are at home," or "Share with me a little about what foods agree with you," in an attempt to assess if the patient is having physical difficulty with eating. Is the patient experiencing tooth pain? Are his dentures ill fitting? Also important to explore are dietary restrictions, faith-based observances, or any cultural norms associated with intake and self-care.

The nurse may also ask whether the patient is hearing voices although the patient may not readily share that information. If so, the nurse will want to try to understand if the voices contribute to lack of self-care. The nurse can also observe the patient for evidence of auditory hallucinations. Behaviors to watch for include talking to oneself or appearing to respond physically to unseen stimuli. This patient may shake his head or cup his hands over the ears as if to protect himself from the voices.

When interacting with a patient who is withdrawn, the nurse must be looking for any changes that may indicate medical complications. Distinct changes in speech patterns, level of attention, and concentration may indicate change in blood sugar. Are vital signs within normal limits? Are pulse and blood pressure low? Does the patient demonstrate orthostatic changes? The nurse will assess lethargy, responsiveness, and changes in gait as indicators of possible dehydration or of untoward side effects of medication such as lithium intoxication or neuroleptic malignant syndrome.

As patients improve, nurses must assess for active self-harm as well. A profoundly depressed patient may often seem lethargic and have slowed thinking, and so the risk for self-harm is not evident. However, nursing staff must ask questions about suicidal ideation and plans. As medical interventions allow for improved sleep and decreased lethargy, the profoundly depressed patient may have the energy to enact a plan of self-harm.

On the unit. Nursing staff must be mindful of cues that patient health or safety is compromised. Does the patient appear dehydrated? Does she appear lethargic? Are there times the patient will eat? Does she tolerate snacks or small packages of food such as breakfast bars or individual boxes of cereal (versus the meal tray, which may be overwhelming)? Will she take in fluids and what type?

With a patient who is profoundly depressed or catatonic, mobility could be impaired. The nurse should assess the patient's extremities for swelling or redness. In addition, he must assess overall skin integrity as a consequence of prolonged immobility.

The patient who is withdrawn may not respond to urges of hunger, thirst, or even need to use the bathroom. Nursing staff must observe further skin turgor and dryness of mouth. Further, staff must watch for incontinence and also monitor skin integrity in order to avoid infection. If the patient is not independently toileting, the nurse should assess urine output and bowel movements. Urine output should be measured and assessed for color as indications of dehydration. The nurse should assess bowel sounds as an indicator of constipation.

● Key Nursing Interventions to Prevent Passive Self-Injury

Provide education and problem-solve. The nurse will offer honest discussion and education about the aspects of treatment the patient is having a hard time engaging in, including difficulty taking food, fluids, or medications. The nurse will approach the patient with a nonjudgmental, problem-solving approach, which conveys her interest in the patient and willingness to understand his thoughts or feelings.

In this manner, she will encourage the patient to share what his barriers are for engagement. She can then work with the patient to find ways to manage these barriers. The nurse may also engage family members in problem solving.

For the patient who is withdrawn and more suspicious of treatment interventions, the information should be imparted in a factual, nonemotional manner. It is important not to push the patient too hard to engage in a certain behavior, or in groups or individual meetings, as this will only seem more threatening, and increase withdrawal. It will be better to offer some basic information such as "I am concerned that you have not been drinking a lot of water, and you need water to be healthy. Have you noticed that you are not drinking a lot?" She may also comment that adequate nutrition and hydration can have a positive effect on mood, energy, and concentration. Then, the nurse can ask if the patient has further questions. If the patient is able to read, then written material may be helpful.

Use prompting. Prompting may also facilitate engagement. The nurse may say, "It is time for breakfast," "Come and have your vital signs done," or "Time to come for morning medication." These informal prompts that are even given globally throughout the unit are less threatening because they simply serve as reminders. For the patient who is extremely withdrawn, prompts may have to take the form of concrete and directive instruction or even direct assistance. These prompts should be directive but gentle: "Take the toothbrush and brush your teeth," "It is time to put on your clean shirt," "Give me your arm so I can take your vital signs," "It is time to get out of bed; sit up and put your feet on the floor."

Make modifications to how food and fluids are typically offered. The withdrawn patient's lack of engagement often encompasses nourishing and hydrating themselves. Offering smaller and more frequent opportunities for intake may be better than only offering food at mealtimes. The nurse can ensure that snacks are nutritionally dense and offer supplemental beverages if solid food seems overwhelming. A sandwich or other handheld food may be less daunting than managing a meal and utensils. For the patient who is paranoid, she may feel more comfortable eating meals brought in by her family or having prepackaged food that she can open herself. Creating an environment where the patient can have the most control and comfort will facilitate not only improved nutritional intake but also improved engagement in treatment more generally. If the patient is taking medication and hydrating only on command, then a regimen for fluid intake should be instituted with a designated target intake. The nurse must communicate with the treatment team about intake and output as medical interventions such as intravenous hydration and parenteral nutrition and/or medication may need to be instituted by the physician.

Assist with using the bathroom and performing basic hygiene. In determining how to intervene with hygiene, the nurse must evaluate what is necessary for the patient to accomplish for health reasons versus what is a cultural norm or expectation but is not absolutely necessary. The nurse may start with prompts for critical hygiene tasks. He may then move to simple commands such as, "Here is a wet facecloth, I need you to wash your face right now." With the catatonic patient who engages in echopraxia, the nurse can mimic the motions of washing one's face to see if the patient will follow along.

If prompts do not work, the nurse must move on to attempting gentle, hands-on assistance. In doing so, the nurse should describe what is being done at each step. For example, she might say, "We are going to change your shirt now, please lift your arms." If the patient has catatonia, care should be delivered by two staff for safety reasons as this patient can display sudden agitated movements.

If difficulties with basic hygiene persist, then partnering with the family could be of benefit. The family may be able to provide certain toiletries the patient prefers. Furthermore, sometimes the patient may allow for more hands-on assistance from a family member than from a stranger.

Encourage acceptance of medication and medical interventions. Medical stabilization is an essential part of treatment, and the entire treatment team must work closely together to ensure patient safety. First, staff must always educate patients about all aspects of medical interventions, that is, the nurse must patiently explain why all patients have routine vital signs, and why a urine or blood sample for lab work may be needed. If the patient has difficulty concentrating and recalling that a urine sample is needed, the nurse can lock the patient's bathroom door with a written reminder on the outside.

Sometimes having a trusted staff member try to engage and impress upon the patient what needs to be done, the importance of the intervention, and the options of how the actions can be completed will move the patient toward participating voluntarily. However, if the risk of compromise to the patient's health is significant, then staff will have to be even more assertive and physically guide the patient toward the appropriate intervention. An example is a patient who is profoundly depressed with psychomotor retardation and does not ambulate to the restroom but urinates on the chair in which she is sitting. For patient safety, staff must now physically guide her and administer care to avoid breakdown in skin integrity and infection.

Patients have the right to refuse medication as long as they do not pose an imminent threat to themselves or others and under these circumstances staff can only use encouragement. It is important to assess the reasons for refusal as these reasons can point to interventions. If the patient is experiencing uncomfortable side effects from medication, then education about the expected duration of the side effects or interventions to diminish specific side effects may be helpful. If the patient is refusing medication because he believes that taking medication signifies weakness or that he could fix his problem if he just tried harder, the nurse may help the patient to challenge this belief. The nurse can offer education about the many causes of mental illness that are beyond the patient's control, such as genetic influences or early childhood experiences. The nurse could compare mental illness to other medical conditions, such as diabetes or hypertension, where medication is a better-understood necessity. This education may begin to take away self-blame and enhance engagement. If the patient has paranoid ideation, opening the medication package in front of him may help. The nurse may also engage family and friends as part of the team to encourage patients to participate in medication treatment.

Patients with profound depression or catatonia may neither verbally agree nor disagree to taking medication but may be unable to coordinate swallowing medication and seem to spit it out. A discussion with the treating physician should include choices around how the medication might be administered. Some options might include sublingual, parenteral, or by injection. When administering this medication, the nurse must continue to talk with the patient about what is happening, the medication they are receiving, and details about how medication will be given. This should be done in an informative way and not a punitive manner. For example, the nurse could say, "I have medication for you. Because you had some problems with swallowing, the doctor would like you to have an injection. The medication is...and I am going to give it to you in your right arm. This medicine should help...If you want to try the kind you swallow please tell me."

● Subgoal: Prevention of Harm to Others

Assessment of Risk for Harm to Others
In report. There are many internal processes that can increase risk for aggression in the patient who is withdrawn. This patient may be unexpectedly aggressive in an attempt to protect himself, as seen in dementia or paranoia. Those with catatonia may suddenly exhibit agitated movement that could be dangerous but perhaps not specifically directed at others. In report, staff may consider the following questions in order to assess risk for aggression:

- Is there an alteration in thought process that is contributing to a misinterpretation of the environment? Does the patient perceive the environment as threatening in some way? Is the patient confused and having difficulty adjusting to changes in the environment?
- Are there any language barriers making it harder to accurately perceive the environment? Do these contribute to increased threat perception?
- How was the patient's behavior during the previous shift? Was he able to be engaged on a one-to-one or group intervention? If not, then what level of intervention was tolerated that allowed for assessment and maintained safety? This is important because pushing a patient beyond where he feels safe may precipitate aggression;
- What is the patient's ability to tolerate assistance with self-care? Or did the patient exhibit sudden agitated movements?

One-to-one contact. If the patient is willing to talk, when deciding on a place to talk, the nurse will be mindful of his personal safety. If checking on the patient in her room, the nurse should maintain at least a leg's length of distance and remain near the door. If sitting during the interaction, the nurse should make sure he always has easy access to the door and that chairs are not directly facing each other. This chair arrangement may be less threatening and may create an opportunity to quickly move away for both the patient and staff. In addition, the nurse will let other staff know that he is checking on a patient in her room so that others are quickly available if needed.

If the patient has been responsive to the interaction, the nurse can try more in-depth evaluation of thought patterns, asking about hallucinations or delusions. If the patient is hearing voices, the nurse will ask the patient directly if the voices are telling her to harm anyone. The nurse can ask, "Are the voices frightening to you?" "Do the voices ever tell you to hurt others?" "Do you feel you must do what the voices are telling you?"

The nurse can explore delusional thinking to determine whether the patient is feeling fearful or threatened. Feelings of being threatened may occur even in the absence of hallucinations or delusional thinking. The nurse should ask the patient about what makes her feel threatened or unsafe in general and what might help her to adjust to being on the unit. By understanding this, nursing staff can work with the patient regarding ways to increase a sense of safety, thus decreasing potential for acting out to protect oneself.

If the nurse asks a question that the patient is not comfortable with, as communicated either verbally or nonverbally, then she should acknowledge to the patient that she notes his increased anxiety or discomfort. Signs of discomfort may include scanning the room, restlessness, diminished eye contact, or muscle tension. If the patient is receptive to the nurse's observation, this can build trust, promote discussion, and avoid aggression. However, if the patient should become guarded, the nurse can express appreciation of the patient's willingness and work in the discussion up until that point and then ask what he would like to do next.

On the unit. Sometimes, a patient who is actively withdrawn can appear to become notably more withdrawn. This may indicate that the patient is escalating and needs to be assessed by the staff. The nurse should keep in mind that any distinct change in presentation warrants further assessment. It is important that nursing staff always be mindful of situations that may become potentially violent. The patient who is experiencing dementia or psychosis will have a limited repertoire of coping skills. The more withdrawn and mute a patient is the more difficult it may be to verbally assess the risk. Careful observation of nonverbal communication becomes essential to planning care and maintaining safety.

● **Key Nursing Interventions for Decreasing Risk of Harm to Others**

Identify triggers for aggression and make a proactive plan for managing them. Whenever possible, the nurse will work with the patient to identify cues or triggers for aggressive behavior. If the patient is mute or does not participate in discussion, the staff should work together to identify triggers for a particular patient. Triggers for aggression are often idiosyncratic but could include another person touching the patient, loud noises, visitors entering the unit, general activity of the milieu, or even the person perceiving their needs as not being met. Throughout this planning process, the nurse will give the constant message that the patient can take control of her behavior at any time. If the patient cannot participate in the planning process, staff may develop their own plan to help the patient avoid what they believe are triggers for aggression for that patient.

Offer assistance when a patient seems agitated. A patient who is more aggressive may feel very isolated. The nurse can remind such a patient that staff is available to help the patient work out a plan to cope with isolation and aggressive feelings. The nurse may say, "It seems like you are having a hard time, let's see what can help," or "I notice you seem upset; how are you doing?" When talking with the person who is more agitated, it is important to be mindful of one's own tone of voice and make sure that it remains calm and gentle, even if the patient begins to yell.

There are several interventions that the nurse can offer to the patient. Please see Chapter 1, "The Patient With Anger," for specific suggestions for a patient who is able to verbally communicate with staff. For the patient who is mute or catatonic, the nurse will need to actively monitor for increased activity and intervene by directing the patient to a safe area or activity.

Provide medications to decrease agitation. As early as possible in the patient's stay on the unit, the nurse should educate the patient about the medications that are available to help the patient calm down and how they are best used. She can encourage the patient to evaluate his own feelings and if possible seek out help through interaction and medication. The nurse should provide simple education to the patient even if he is mute. If the patient is not able to identify the need for intervention, and agitation is elevated, then staff needs to take a gentle and supportive but firm approach. The nurse may let the patient know that it appears he is having a difficult time and that medication may help. Benzodiazepines and atypical antipsychotics have been useful in treating catatonia and may be ordered for this patient. Please see also Chapter 12, "Medication Administration."

Containment. In the event that a patient is increasingly agitated and at imminent risk for harm to self or others, and that all other interventions are not successful, the staff may make the decision to contain the patient. Please refer to Chapter 7, "The Patient With Paranoia."

TREATMENT ENGAGEMENT AND STABILIZATION

● **Subgoal: Help Patient to Decrease Withdrawal and Increase Treatment Engagement**

Assessment of Ability to Engage in Treatment

In report. During report, staff should begin to build a collective picture of the patient's current ability to engage in the milieu. The initial report from the admission should have relevant data such as level of functioning prior to admission, highest level of functioning in the past year, as well as intellectual and developmental levels. It is also important to know if English is this patient's primary language. This knowledge will help the staff to identify realistic goals for engagement.

In shift-to-shift report, staff should share specific details regarding the patient's type of withdrawal (passive or active) in particular situations, level of engagement, response to different types of interventions, and response to medication on the previous shift. In particular, how did the patient take medications? What was the response? For some patients with catatonia, a dose of lorazepam can have a remarkable beneficial effect allowing the patient to be able to eat, move independently, and interact with others. What groups did the patient attend? Did he eat spontaneously? Did the patient wash or change his clothing independently or with less prompting?

One-to-one contact. Throughout the one-to-one contact, the nurse should assess for the verbal and nonverbal cues given by the patient that contact is tolerable or not. If contact seems tolerable, the nurse can slowly begin to ask questions that may give some insight into what the patient can tolerate and the reasons for withdrawal. Reasons for withdrawal that the patient may be able to articulate and that the nurse may ask about include intense emotions such as anxiety, sadness, frustration, or shame; hallucinations or delusions; or beliefs that treatment will not be helpful or is not necessary. Even if the patient cannot articulate reasons for withdrawal directly in response to questioning, as the nurse talks to the patient, he may note relevant themes in the patient's speech. For example, if the patient states, "Nothing is going to get better," then staff can hypothesize that hopelessness and sadness are related to withdrawal. For the eating disordered patient who refuses to consume dinner because "you just want to make me fat," nursing staff can understand they are frightened and angry.

The patient may not be able to articulate reasons for withdrawal if it is due to dementia, delirium, or catatonia. For these patients, the nurse may have to place the priority on treatment engagement rather than on assessment of underlying thought patterns or reasons for withdrawal. If the patient is able to converse, the topic of the conversation may stay on a "light" level. The nurse can, however, listen carefully to what the patient says to see if there are any signs of cognitive difficulties or confusion.

On the unit. When on the unit, both the actively and passively withdrawn patient should be observed for how he tolerates different levels of stimuli. What is his proximity to others? Does he respond to brief but frequent observation or interaction from staff such as in unit checks? Does he respond more to males or females? Is the patient responsive to directive intervention? When a pattern develops, nursing staff can use this information to develop interventions at the level the patient can tolerate.

● Key Nursing Interventions to Decrease Withdrawal and Increase Treatment Engagement

Communicate in ways that increase engagement. Breeze and Repper (1998) conducted focus groups with nurses and patients in order to understand most effective interventions for "difficult" patients. From this research, it was clear that approaching the patient with a supportive stance was more effective than approaching the patient with a controlling stance. Therefore, the nurse will keep the following principles in mind when interacting with patients who are withdrawn, including but not limited to one-to-one contacts. These principles will increase the chances of engagement, as well as serve to help avoid aggression or further withdrawal. The nurse will

- Make brief but frequent contact or sit quietly with a patient for brief time periods
- Consider having casual meeting times rather than planned and structured meetings, as the casual meetings may be less threatening
- Allow the patient to refuse contact or refuse interventions
- Ask the patient for permission to talk together
- Allow the patient to choose the location of the interaction or of an activity
- Consider creative ways to engage in interaction. For example, doing a craft together or just sitting quietly with a patient. Interactions may occur in the context of giving medications, eating, or completing activities of daily living
- Strive for consistency in the staff who interact with the patient. Consistency in care will reduce stimuli for the patient and allow him to have better focus. Also, with consistency there is more possibility for the patient to develop trust in staff members
- Make sure to not overwhelm the person with too many questions trying to assess how she is. This may cause further withdrawal. It is better to say, "how are you doing today?" and let the patient guide the verbal exchange. If the patient has very little to say, then the nurse may move on to guide the patient in health maintenance activities.

For example, he may say, "Let me walk you over to the kitchen for breakfast"

- Allow adequate time for the patient who is withdrawn to process the verbal input from the nurse and then organize his thoughts to give a response. The nurse may be thinking more quickly than the patient who is withdrawn. Because it is important to provide undivided attention to the patient, the nurse will need to focus and not allow her mind to wander

The nurse will often begin an interaction with the patient who is withdrawn on a nonthreatening level, discussing commonly relatable topics, such as hobbies, movies, or other social topics. Nonthreatening topics give rich insight into the likes and dislikes of the patient, as well as areas in which he may feel resourceful. Once the patient appears a bit more comfortable, has a connection with the nurse, and has had a chance to talk about the hospital experience in general, the nurse may turn to more in-depth questions.

Throughout, the nurse will keep in mind that validating feelings expressed without judgment is a foundation for interpersonal engagement. He will make efforts to allow the patient to feel that she is accepted. He will try to communicate that the patient's safety and well-being are the highest priority.

Be conscious of verbal and nonverbal communication with mute patients. For the patient who is profoundly withdrawn and nonresponsive, as in catatonia, dementia, or depression, the nurse still avails himself to the patient on regular intervals throughout the shift. He will continue to verbalize to the patient that he is going to sit with her for a while, help her eat, or help with other activities. The nurse will talk to this patient as if she is going to respond but without overwhelming her with speech. The nurse should ask only one question at a time and allow for sufficient time for the patient to process the question, develop an answer, and verbally respond (even if the patient does not respond). The nurse can also simply tell the patient what the nurse is going to do and then sit quietly. Sitting quietly with a person conveys she is important and that the nurse cares. The nurse should keep in mind that it is not good clinical care for staff to have conversations with one another as if the patient could not hear them, as it depersonalizes the patient and may disengage her further.

Choose appropriate groups and/or unit activities. Having numerous activities that meet the needs of patients at different levels of care is very important when engaging patients in treatment. If a patient feels overwhelmed by a particular activity, this may foster increased withdrawal. The nurse and patient should try to find the appropriate level of activity for the patient so that the patient can experience success. For some patients, such as the patient with dementia, success may be tolerating the activity of the unit without agitation. For another patient, sitting on the periphery of a group and listening to others will be a treatment goal. The nurse can encourage the patient to do this by saying, "I know you are not ready to talk in group, but sometimes it is helpful to hear how others are working through their illness." For another patient, being able to sit and share mealtime with others may be a significant stride toward engagement. Staff should praise patients for small successes in various activities; this can foster self-confidence for the patient and further engagement in treatment.

Provide interventions that decrease anxiety. As discussed above, for some patients, withdrawal may be related to high levels of anxiety. Decreasing anxiety may lead to increased ability to engage in treatment. Please see Chapter 2, "The Patient With Anxiety," for strategies for helping patients to cope with anxiety.

Treat underlying conditions. Delirium, psychotic processes, or medical illnesses may underlie withdrawal. With any of these conditions, the role of the nurse will be to monitor the physical health of the patient and report significant findings to the treating physician. In addition, the nurse will administer medications and monitor the patient's response. Finally, the nurse will also provide education to the patient about his underlying condition, using the language that the patient can understand. Please also see Chapter 7, "The Patient With Paranoia" for strategies on working with patients with paranoia.

Help to increase motivation for treatment. Some patients who are actively withdrawn and refusing treatment do so because they believe treatment is unnecessary. These patients may include those with eating disorders, mania, nonsuicidal self-injury, or substance-use disorders. If a patient believes treatment is unnecessary or has been forced into it, the nurse's role is to provide support for the patient and help her to explore her ambivalence about treatment. The nurse will listen for any indication that the patient sees any benefits to treatment and will explore these perceived benefits further with the patient. Please see Chapter 4, "The Patient With Manic Behavior" and Chapter 8, "The Patient With Substance Use Disorders" for further strategies for increasing acceptance of and motivation for treatment.

PREPARATION FOR DISCHARGE

Discharge planning should focus on supporting this patient's continued engagement in treatment and in the environment when he returns home. Establishing post-discharge appointments and discussing methods with the patient for remembering those appointments (e.g., keeping a calendar) will be helpful. It will be important to engaging community resources, such as community mental health centers or group therapy opportunities. An active discussion with the patient regarding the use of these resources will be an important educational opportunity. Finally, the nurse can work with the patient to review the reasons for withdrawal, the patient's progress over time while on the inpatient unit, and what interventions or activities may have helped the patient progress. If the patient gives permission, it will be very useful to engage the patient's family in preparation for discharge.

TABLE 10.1
Goals, Areas of Assessment, and Interventions for a Patient
Who is Withdrawn

Goal	Assessment	Intervention
	Safety	
Prevent passive self-harm	Review medical history Assess nutrition, hydration, self-care, acceptance of medications, and mobility Try to understand reasons why the patient is refusing care Assess for behavioral changes that may indicate medical complications As patient improves, assess for active self-harm ideation or behavior	Provide education and problem-solving Use prompting Make modifications to how food and fluids are typically offered Assist with using the bathroom and performing basic hygiene Encourage acceptance of medication and medical interventions
Prevent harm to others	Assess internal processes that can increase risk for aggression, such as fear related to believing that the environment is threatening in some way Note patient's previous pattern of aggressive behavior Watch for distinct changes in presentation	Identify triggers for aggression and make a proactive plan for managing them Offer assistance when a patient seems agitated Provide medications to decrease agitation

(cont.)

TABLE 10.1
Goals, Areas of Assessment, and Interventions for a Patient
Who is Withdrawn *(cont.)*

Goal	Assessment	Intervention
Stabilization and Engagement		
Help patient to decrease withdrawal and increase treatment engagement	Review functioning prior to the episode precipitating hospitalization Assess effect of treatments on engagement Try to understand reasons for withdrawal Watch the patient's ability to engage in activities on the unit	Communicate in ways that increase engagement Be conscious of verbal and nonverbal communication with mute patients Choose appropriate groups and/or unit activities Provide interventions to decrease anxiety Treat underlying conditions Help increase motivation for treatment

Note: A PDF containing all ten of the tables from Section I is available for free download and convenient printing from springerpub.com/Damon

REFERENCES

Breeze, J., & Repper, J. (1998). Struggling for control: The care experiences of 'difficult' patients in mental health services. *Journal of Advanced Nursing, 28*(6), 1301–1311.

DeNuccio, G., & Schwartz-Barcott, D. (2000). A concept analysis of withdrawal: Application of the hybrid model. In B. Rodgers, & K. Knafl (Eds.), *Concept development in nursing* (pp. 161–192). Philadelphia, PA: Saunders.

Fortinash, K. M., & Holoday-Worret, P. A. (2008). *Psychiatric mental health nursing* (4th ed.). St. Louis, MO: Mosby Elsevier.

Penland, H. R., Weder, N., & Tampi, R. R. (2006). The catatonic dilemma expanded. *Annals of General Psychiatry, 5*(14), 1–9. doi: 10.1186/1744-859X-5-14

Townsend, M. C. (2008). *Essentials of psychiatric mental health nursing: Concepts of care in evidence-based practice* (4th ed.). Philadelphia, PA: F.A. Davis Company.

Varcarolis, E. M., & Halter, M. J. (2010). *Foundations of psychiatric mental health nursing: A clinical approach* (6th ed.). St Louis, MO: Saunders Elsevier.

Videbeck, S. L. (2011). *Psychiatric-mental health nursing* (5th ed.). Philadelphia, PA: Wolters Kluwer/Lippincott Williams & Wilkins.

Family Interventions

Michelle Pereira and Judy L. Sheehan

11

INTRODUCTION

The importance of engaging families of patients with psychiatric illness in the hospitalization process has been acknowledged for decades. Still, research suggests that in general, family members of patients who have experienced at least one or more inpatient psychiatric hospitalizations express great dissatisfaction with their involvement and interactions with staff (Hanson, 1995). Effective change can only be brought about if nurses and other medical personnel make a conscious effort to understand the family perspective and emotions involved with a loved one's psychiatric hospitalization. How a family member copes with hospitalization is affected by concerns about stigma, previous experiences, and strong emotions—particularly fear. In some cases, previous encounters with the mental health system may have imparted feelings of frustration; other families may be harboring guilt about their family member's illness. To succeed in effectively engaging family members, the nurse must recognize the family's need for acceptance, desire to be included, and the power of hope.

THE EXPERIENCE OF THE FAMILY

Stigma Associated With Psychiatric Illness

Despite efforts by organizations worldwide to eliminate the stigma attached to psychiatric illness, society has been slow to react. The public often treats patients with psychiatric illness differently as compared to any other group of medical patients. Even groups involved in the care of people with psychiatric illness do not always have attitudes toward these patients that are as positive as one would expect (Lauber & Sartorius, 2007). The segregation and neglect experienced by individuals who suffer from psychiatric disorders is often experienced by their family members as well (Lauber & Sartorius, 2007). At the very least, social rejection of the person with psychiatric illness translates into a tremendous stress on the caretakers and families of the patient (Lauber & Sartorius, 2007). Most family members do not believe that others avoid them because of a relative's hospitalization, whereas many do report concealing this information to at least some degree (Phelan, Bromet, & Link, 1998). Fear of stigma can affect family attitudes and behavior regarding the hospitalization experience; families may feel resentment and even anger toward the patient.

Family's Reactions to Inpatient Hospitalization

Many families describe the experience of hospitalization as being filled with mixed emotions; on the one hand, they feel relief and are grateful for help, but on the other hand, they also feel a sense of loss and guilt (Hanson, 1995). This guilt arises because family members feel as though they are simply abandoning their loved one by seeking professional help (Hanson, 1995). They may also feel anxiety, fear, resentment, hopelessness, and helplessness. In addition to experiencing these intense emotions, families are subject to an abrupt physical and emotional cutoff from their family member when she is admitted. Further, after admission, family members report feeling excluded from any significant information about what is happening with their loved one and hopeless in dealing with mental health professionals (Hanson, 1995).

As a result of these mixed and intense emotions, and of feeling excluded from what is happening, family members may act angrily toward the nurse or each other. The nurse may witness family members arguing and yelling at one another or even experience a family member shouting out demands concerning the care of his relative. How the nurse responds is integral to how the family members will continue to interact with one another, the hospitalized relative, and those to whom they have entrusted the care of their relative. While these situations may be frustrating, it is important for the nurse to remember how difficult this experience is for the family and to act with compassion. Nurses should anticipate that these situations will occur.

STRATEGIES TO EFFECTIVELY ENGAGE FAMILY MEMBERS

Use Good Communication Skills

Psychiatric nurses will strive to develop a dialogue with families that will convey a genuine concern for the patient *and* the family. In talking with the family, the nurse should keep in mind that it is not uncommon for family members to experience difficulty in asking questions or not to know what questions to ask. It is important for the nurse to employ communication skills that will help put family members at ease in order that underlying issues provoking increased anxiety may be addressed. Effective communication skills include the following:

- *Attentive listening.* This includes making good eye contact, listening to the family members' concerns, conveying empathy and acceptance of difficult emotions, asking pertinent open-ended questions, allowing for silence in the conversation, and asking for feedback.
- *Paraphrasing.* Using paraphrasing, the nurse will restate in his own words what he believes to be the essential content communicated by a family member. This

demonstrates to the family member that the nurse has heard and understood what the family member is saying. If the nurse has not interpreted the family member correctly, paraphrasing offers an opportunity for clarification by the family member. For example, a family member may say, "Manuela has been so depressed—I try to help with the kids, cleaning, and shopping—it's hard—school is starting—I'll have to work around that schedule, get some time at the office and still be here for Manuela." The nurse may paraphrase this by saying "You have many demands upon you right now."

- *Reflecting feelings.* In reflection, the nurse tries to clarify and restate what the family member is saying. Effective use of reflection may (1) increase the nurse's understanding of the other family member, (2) help the family member to clarify his thoughts, and (3) reassure the family member that someone is willing to attend to his point of view and wants to help. Reflection is similar to paraphrasing, but rather than restating back the content, it reflects back the *feeling* being communicated in the message. For example, when the family member says, "Manuela has been so depressed—I try to help with the kids, cleaning and shopping—it's hard—school is starting—I'll have to work around that schedule, get some time at the office and still be here for Manuela," the nurse may say, "You're feeling overwhelmed right now."

React to Anger With a Nondefensive Stance

In some cases, a family member may seem angry with the nurse for their loved one's situation. A family member might have good reason to be angry—there could be necessary redirection of resources to the ill family member or interference with significant family events (graduations, weddings, funerals, etc.). It is important that the nurse allow emotionally charged family members to express themselves to better understand their perspective.

The nurse might ask about previous psychiatric hospital experiences. If those experiences were negative, the nurse should find out why the family was dissatisfied in the past and ask what specific things he could do to make the experience better.

Welcome Information From Family Members

Spouses and parents often want to get involved at an early stage and may have a need to express opinions and past experiences. While the family may view the nurse as having clinical expertise, they likewise may (correctly) view themselves as having expert knowledge of the hospitalized family member. Recognizing the family as a resource allows the nurse to receive information essential to the patient's treatment and recovery.

Provide Family Members With Information Tailored to What They Need

Family members have strong need for information. It is important to provide the family with as much information as possible. However, it is equally important to adjust and individualize information; nurses must be aware that flooding family members with information may actually increase anxiety and decrease the family member's ability to hear and focus on essential points. Therefore, in order to effectively share information, the nurse should adjust the amount of information according to what the family needs or can tolerate, repeat information as necessary, and allow time for questions.

Provide Hope to Family Members

One of the most important things a nurse can do is providing hope for the family of patients with psychiatric illness. Engaging family members in meaningful dialogue is an opportunity for the nurse to instill hope. Families need to be reassured and reminded that by undergoing treatment, the patient is making strides toward a healthier future. Nurses should ask about family expectations and their goals for their loved one both during *and after* hospitalization. Hope is not only essential to the patient's well being but also important for increasing a family member's ability to cope with the current situation and plan for the future.

CONFIDENTIALITY

One of the biggest challenges in communicating with families is navigating around the rules regarding confidentiality. In order for nurses to be able to disclose personal information about any patient over the age of 18, written consent must be received from the patient. Sometimes, patients feel embarrassed or, for some other reason, do not wish to grant family members the access to any specific information during hospitalization. Typically, families do not expect confidentiality to be a barrier in communicating with staff and are therefore taken aback if it does become one (Marshall & Solomon, 2003). This can extremely upset the families and even evoke strong feelings of resentment and anger towards the treatment team staff.

To help avoid these situations, nurses should discuss and provide an outline of the procedures for releasing information to families shortly after admission of the patient (Marshall & Solomon, 2003). The nurse can also note that even if a patient chooses to withhold confidential information, the nurse is still allowed to provide general information about psychiatric illness and that receiving information from families is not against confidentiality rules (Marshall & Solomon, 2003).

If a family member does inquire about a patient who has decided not to disclose information to her family, the nurse should not simply dismiss family questions. Instead, the nurse should make time to explain to families that the decision to withhold confidential information is made by the patient, and that staff does not make the decision for patients. Although it seems simple, this may help ease some of the tension that arises between families and staff.

FURTHER SUPPORT AND INFORMATION FOR FAMILIES

Support Groups

Nurses can further improve the experience of families by pointing them to various resources and support groups. The National Alliance on Mental Illness (NAMI) sponsors a free, twelve-week program known as the Family-to-Family Education Program. This program has been shown to successfully diminish worry within family members (Dixon et al., 2001). In weekly sessions, caregivers receive information about mental illnesses and common treatments, while developing effective problem solving and communication strategies (NAMI, 2011). The program is a way for families to stay involved even if their loved one chooses not to disclose specific information.

Mental Health Law

Although specific parameters vary from state to state, the mental health law guides the practices of any psychiatric facility, including protocols for discharge and release of patient information. Becoming familiar with the mental health law can be very beneficial for family members of patients, especially those experiencing hospitalization for the first time.

PRACTICAL INFORMATION FOR INTERACTING WITH FAMILIES IN PARTICULAR SITUATIONS

Admissions

Patients and family members experience many conflicting and intense emotions at the time of admissions, and family members may have many concerns. Therefore, when a patient is admitted, it is helpful if the nurse can talk with the family and specifically address any concerns the family may have. The nurse can provide general information about the unit, including the names of the members of the treatment team along with their roles and visiting hours. Two other important issues to discuss are the rights of psychiatric patients (including confidentiality) and safety concerns.

General information about the unit. It is important for families to understand exactly what the roles are for different members of the treatment team, such as nurses, social workers, and physicians. This can help eliminate confusion about to whom certain questions should be directed. In helping to improve the experience of family members of patients, a nurse should be sure that contact information for relevant providers is accurate, accessible, and printed for the family. This information should also include best times for the family to make contact. The nurse should also include written information about the timing of visiting hours and any guidelines about visiting hours.

Rights of psychiatric patients. Family members can forget that their loved one is entering a hospital designed to provide care. Families may fear that once in a facility, patients will be treated unfairly or with force. The psychiatric nurse can ease these fears. Family members will benefit greatly from a simple reminder of the overarching principle guiding the behavior and attitudes of all staff. Employees within the psychiatric hospital have chosen to dedicate their lives to provide helping care for others and are there to improve patients' quality of life. Nurses should place special emphasis on the rights of the patient within a facility. For example, it may help families to know that medication is taken by choice. Nurses should also provide an overview of the confidentiality rights of patients, as described above.

Safety concerns. One of the biggest concerns facing family members of any psychiatric patient is safety. Upon hospitalization, families will often question, "Is my loved one in danger?" and "Who is in charge of making sure they are safe?" The nurse should reassure families that their loved one will be safe throughout the duration of her stay. Family members may express concern not only about their relative but also about the behaviors of other patients on the unit. Family members may wonder if the other patients might steal personal belongings, enter their family member's room uninvited, or otherwise harm their family member. A brief overview of the inpatient environment, the process and frequency by which the staff monitor the safety of patients, and the initial plan of treatment may help put the family at ease.

A major concern of families of geriatric patients is that their loved one may fall. The nurse should make time to explain to the family the precautionary actions hospital staff take to help reduce this risk. Strategies may differ slightly from facility to facility, but most hospitals complete a fall-risk assessment upon admission. The assessment allows nurses and other staff to increase vigilance and take more precautions for those patients with a greater fall risk. Being familiar with some of the actions taken to reduce falls will help ease family worries and stress.

Upon hospitalization of a suicidal patient, family members need reassurance that their loved one will be protected from hurting himself. Families will worry that potentially dangerous objects will be accessible to their relative. The nurse should take time to explain specific measures, taken on the unit where their loved one will be staying, designed to reduce the risk of patients inflicting self-harm. It will help if the family also understands that once admitted to the hospital, patients enter a treatment plan that usually consists of pharmacotherapy and psychotherapy. When the plan is followed and the patient is carefully monitored, the risk of a patient attempting suicide dramatically decreases.

OVER THE TELEPHONE

Family members may want to call (sometimes frequently) to check on the progress and well-being of their relative. As soon as possible, the nurse should provide in writing all relevant staff contacts and telephone numbers to the family member. The nurse may also want to identify a particular staff contact and establish a specific check-in time for the family member. The nurse can advise the family member to write her questions or concerns down before calling in order to ensure that they are addressed during the call. This strategy often discourages multiple calls on the part of the family member and improves communication.

Phone calls can be very difficult when patients do not want any disclosure by their treatment team to their family members. The nurse must be firm but kind with the family member. One potential way to partially address this is for the nurse to discuss the caller's concern with the patient and ask the patient to call the family member to discuss that concern or to give the nurse permission to call.

Visiting Hours

Having printed material on hand informing the family about visiting hours will help the family in organizing their daily schedules. There may be instances when a family member cannot visit during regular hours, and the nurse should make reasonable effort to accommodate special circumstances.

Objects brought to patients during visiting hours. Visiting hours provide an opportunity for family members to bring their relative cosmetics, food, cell phones, and other items of comfort from home. Staff should be aware of the items brought in to the patient and should ensure that those items fall within acceptable hospital-safety standards. Family members may not be aware that certain items would be considered a hazard or even contraband within the hospital. Therefore, nurses must be proactive—it is best to provide a list of what family members may or may not bring in to their loved one. This can eliminate an uncomfortable confrontation later. It may help if the nurses explain why some seemingly common items are considered safety hazards on an inpatient psychiatric unit.

Families who are disruptive during visiting hours. Situations may arise during visiting hours in which the family members become disruptive to the functioning of the unit. These situations may include angry outbursts, loud interactions, arguments, demands made of the staff, and crying. Regardless of the situation, the nurse will need to address the matter. He can speak to the disruptive or upset family member and query the cause of the distress. For example, the nurse might say, "I am sorry you are upset. I would like to understand the situation and try to help you." He will attentively listen to the problem and paraphrase the problem to insure he understands it. He may offer compassionate understanding to the family member, for example, by saying "I can understand how you might feel upset." The nurse can then begin to explore options for resolution. He may ask, "How might I help you?" If the situation can be resolved easily, the nurse will do so. If the situation needs to be brought to a higher level, the nurse can call a supervisor or provide a name and phone number for the person to call in the morning. If the situation continues to escalate or if the nurse begins to feel it may become dangerous, he should politely ask the family member to leave the unit. The nurse can call security if the situation escalates quickly. He should also understand the organizational policy for the circumstances in which the local police should be contacted.

Family Meetings

Families will often come in to the hospital for formal meetings with the treatment team. Before a discussion begins, it is important to have a private area set aside for the meeting. This will prevent family members from feeling uncomfortable or worrying about being overheard. Some organizations have nurses involved in family meetings; some do not. Regardless of whether the nurse is involved in the family meeting, the nurse should assess the impact of the meeting on the patient. The nurse should check in with the patient to discuss any concerns before the meeting and then debriefing the patient after the meeting to determine his response. This is one way to ensure that patient needs are identified and staff can provide supportive interventions.

Discharge

The exit meeting provides a forum to review the posthospital treatment plan and provide the patient and the family an opportunity to discuss any lingering fears or concerns about discharge. If, according to organizational policy and procedure, the nurse is able to discuss the treatment plan with the family, this can eliminate some of the anxiety and stress they experience.

Safety after discharge. Perhaps the biggest cause of concern for family members is the safety of their loved one after discharge. Family members become worried about how they will care for the patient and fear that they lack the skills necessary to help prevent a suicide attempt (Sun & Long, 2007). The nurse can provide families with effective strategies and ways to support this patient and help avoid suicidal behaviors. First, she can tell the family that the most important thing a relative or caregiver can do is to create a safe and nurturing environment (Sun & Long, 2007). Although a simple strategy, reminding family members to encourage the expression of feelings and to make themselves available to listen to a patient can help to reduce suicidal behavior (Sun & Long, 2007). Second, prior to discharge, the nurse should ask family members to remove any firearms or weaponry from the house and possibly to lock medicines away. Third, nurses should tell families to be sensitive and watchful for verbal cues from the patient such as statements like "I want to die" (Sun & Long, 2007).

Family members may also fear that violence could occur after discharge, especially if violence was a precursor to hospitalization and the patient discontinues medication after hospitalization. Nurses need to reassure families that discharge only occurs after the treatment team agrees that a patient poses no danger to herself or others. Further, because this is not a guarantee, the nurse should ensure that families not only know what signs and symptoms to look for, but how to get help in determining whether their relative continues to be compliant with treatment.

Family members' roles in continued healing. Family members can take an active role in helping their loved one to heal, and nurses can facilitate family members' understanding on how they may help. In addition to the strategies discussed above, a family member may assist the patient in planning daily activities and discourage long periods of inactivity (Sun & Long, 2007). Further, families can encourage adherence to the treatment plan and to medication regimens (Sun & Long, 2007).

WORKING WITH SPECIFIC TYPES OF FAMILY MEMBERS

Parents. The hospitalization of a young adult may be particularly difficult for the family. Information given to the parents may be limited due to the legal age of the child. The parents, who may be accustomed to high levels of involvement, may feel excluded and disenfranchised. Young adults may need assistance understanding their new role as a legal adult as may not be aware of mental health law or the legal restrictions on sharing information with the parents. In addition, the parents may blame themselves for the illness the patient is experiencing or be embarrassed by the behaviors demonstrated. Parents may feel scared and even ashamed of having a child enter a facility. In many instances, parents expect to be blamed upon hospitalizing their child; this can result in an avoidance of staff interaction (Scharer, 2002). For all of these reasons, it may fall to the nurse to initiate contact with parents who are present at the time of hospitalization, explain relevant rules around confidentiality to all parties, and, if acceptable to the patient, invite parents to participate in the treatment process.

Children of patients. Visits by children to psychiatric inpatient units may warrant special attention by the nursing staff. Depending upon the age and behavior of the child, the nurse may be concerned about the safety of the child and the impact upon the other patients and the milieu. Prior to the visit, the nurse or other treatment team member should have a discussion with the patient and the adult members of the family to determine what the best approach might be. What is the reason for the visit? Has it been determined to be therapeutic by the treatment team? How has the child been prepared for the visit? (O'Brien et al., 2011.) If a conference room is available, it might be reasonable to have the patient and her family spend time together in this more private area. If the child becomes noisy or disruptive on the unit or other patients seem to become distressed, the nurse may need to ask the nonpatient adult to remove the child from the unit for some period of time.

REFERENCES

Dixon, L., Stewart B., Burland, J., Delahanty, J., Lucksted, A., & Hoffman, M. (2001). Pilot study of the effectiveness of the family-to-family education program. *Psychiatric Services, 52,* 965–967.

Hanson, J. G. (1995). Families' perceptions of psychiatric hospital-ization of relatives with a severe mental illness. *Administration and Policy in Mental Health, 22*, 531–541.

Lauber, C., & Sartorius, N. (2007). At issue: Anti-stigma endeavours. *International Review of Psychiatry, 19*, 103–106.

Marshall, T., & Solomon, P. (2003). Professional's responsibility in releasing information to families of adults with mental illness. *Psychiatric Services, 54*, 1622–1628.

National Alliance on Mental Illness. (2011). NAMI family to fam-ily [online] Retrieved from http://www.nami.org/Template.cfm?Section=Family-to-Family

O'Brien, L., Anand, M., Brady, P., & Gillies, D. (2011). Children vis-iting parents in inpatient psychiatric facilities: Perspectives of parents, carers and children. *International Journal of Mental Health Nursing, 20*, 137–143.

Phelan, J. C., Bromet, E. J., & Link, B. G. (1998). Psychiatric illness and family stigma. *Schizophrenia Bulletin, 24*, 115–126.

Sun, F., & Long, A. (2007). A theory to guide families and carers of people who are at risk of suicide. *Journal of Clinical Nursing, 17*, 1939–1948.

Medication Administration

12

Judy L. Sheehan and Joanne M. Matthew

NURSING KNOWLEDGE BASE REGARDING PSYCHIATRIC MEDICATIONS

Medication is an important component of psychiatric mental health treatment. On the psychiatric inpatient unit, nurses are responsible for administering psychiatric medications. However, medication administration is not the single act of having a patient accept a medication from a nurse. Instead, medication administration involves

- Observing a patient's response to medications
- Evaluating the overall effectiveness of medication on target symptoms
- Monitoring any side effects or complications that may arise
- Promptly reporting any important observations to the prescribing clinician

In order to be able to assess efficacy and monitor for side effects, knowledge regarding medications used to treat psychiatric illness is essential. One strategy for thinking about medications is to categorize the type of medication as it applies to various symptoms associated with psychiatric diagnoses.

- Psychotic symptoms such as racing thoughts, thought blocking, disorganized thought processes, delusions, or hallucinations are usually treated with antipsychotic medicine

- Depression symptoms such as anhedonia, pervasive or overwhelming sadness, guilt, and disturbances of sleep, appetite, and energy are often treated with an antidepressant medication
- Bipolar disorder is often treated with a mood stabilizer or antiseizure medication. Depending on the patient's symptoms, other medications may be prescribed as well
- Anxiety symptoms such as intense worrying or panic attacks are treated with certain antidepressants and sometimes benzodiazepines

By understanding the anticipated action of these general classes of psychiatric medications, along with usual dosing patterns and potential side effects or complications, the nurse can generally anticipate patient needs, be watchful for dangerous situations, and report critical information to the treatment team.

This does not, however, remove the responsibility from a nurse to be well informed about any particular psychiatric or nonpsychiatric medication being given to a patient. Because nurses administer medication to patients as a standard part of practice, there is an underlying responsibility to be aware of not only the names of medications but also the mechanism of action, dosages, potential side effects, and possible complications of specific medications administered. New medications, new uses for old medication, and new delivery mechanisms require nurses to continually update their knowledge of psychopharmacology. If the nurse is unfamiliar with a medication, she has a variety of resources available, including drug reference books specifically for nurses, online databases, and product inserts. In addition, the pharmacist is usually able to answer any additional questions that may arise.

ADMINISTERING MEDICATIONS

Right patient–right medication. Psychiatric patients often dress in street clothes and ambulate freely around the inpatient unit. Sometimes, patients may resemble other patients, and it is not unusual to have patients changing clothes frequently throughout the day. Patient identification bands may be removed or become illegible over time, so nurses must have a plan to use patient identifiers when administering medications and should be clear about their agency guidelines regarding this issue. Potential plans may include having photographs available when distributing medications, checking patient bands daily to ensure legibility and replacing them as often as needed, or asking the patient for her name and date of birth (WHO, Collaborating Centre for Patient Safety Solutions, 2007). The medications given on a psychiatric unit are usually tailored to specific patients for very specific reasons. Understanding the reason a particular medication has been ordered for a particular patient will help the nurse ensure the correct medication is delivered to the correct patient. For example, sometimes a medication is selected because its effects will be helpful to the patient (e.g., weight loss or gain, sedation, or stimulation) or the side effect of one medication (e.g., dry mouth) is more tolerable to the patient than a different side effect (e.g., nausea).

Right route–right time–right dose. Psychotropic medication comes in many forms, including pill, liquid, sublingual and injectable, and the absorption rate of the medication will be influenced by the route. An awareness of the absorption rate of a medicine will allow the nurse to anticipate when the patient may begin to feel its effect. A pill will be absorbed more slowly than a liquid, sublingual, or injectable form (Janda & Fagan, 2010). It usually takes 30 to 45 minutes for a patient to feel the effects of oral medications delivered in pill form. Crisis situations will most likely require a liquid concentrate or an inject-able medication in order to address the time sensitive nature of the situation.

The timing of a dose may be influenced by instruc-tions from the prescriber, agency policy and procedures, patient preference, or requirements of the medication itself. Some medications must be given at mealtimes or prior to sleep. The route of a medication may also deter-mine the timing. For example, a sublingual medication must not be given at mealtimes or at the same time as other medications.

Usually, prescribers want to use the least amount of medication necessary to treat a problem. Therefore, they often slowly increase the dose of a medication (i.e., titrate the medication) until symptoms are under control. For example, the prescriber may start a medication as a small standing dose but also order a "prn" medication. If the standing dose is given and the prn is also needed, the phy-sician may use this information to increase the standing dose so that prn medication is not necessary. Although the physicians determine the dosage to be ordered, it will be important for the nurse to provide feedback to the physi-cian regarding the patient's response to the dose and to changes in dosage.

COMMON SIDE EFFECTS AND ADVERSE REACTIONS

Common side effects. Common side effects of psychotro-pic medication may include headache, nausea, weight gain, increased appetite, stomach pain and diarrhea, dizzi-ness, sedation, somnolence, and orthostatic hypotension. Psychoactive medications have been identified to increase the risk of fall for patients of all ages. The nurse should carry out a careful assessment of fall risk, hydration status (via laboratory findings as well as observation of intake), and orthostatic hypotension regularly (Sherrod, Collins, Wynn, & Gragg, 2010). There should be a clear follow-up plan to prevent falls and fall-related injuries for those found to be at risk.

Another type of side effect is extra pyramidal symptoms. Extra pyramidal side effects (EPS) are due to dopamine blockade in the nigrostriatal pathway that is a part of the extra pyramidal system in the brain (Stahl, 2000). Extra pyramidal symptoms include:

- Acute dystonic reaction. This is a sudden severe prolonged muscle contraction involving one or more muscles. Ninety percent of these reactions occur within 4 days after any treatment with an antipsychotic medication, and the most common area these reactions occur is in the muscles of the head and neck (Stanilla & Simpson, 2009). Oculogyric crisis, which involves the eyes shifting upward, is an example of a dystonic reaction
- Akasthisia. Akasthisia means "inability to sit." The patient will have increased activity and a subjective feeling of restlessness (Stanilla & Simpson, 2009)
- Neuroleptic-induced Parkinsonism. Neuroleptic-induced Parkinsonism symptoms can include resting tremor, muscle rigidity, shuffling gait, stooped posture, blunted facial expression, and drooling (Kamin et al., 2000)
- Tardive dyskinesia. This is characterized by the involuntary irregular movement involving muscles of the head, limbs, or trunk. This is a more difficult side effect to manage, and the physician will need to determine treatment options (Howland, 2011)

If the nurse sees signs of EPS, he should report it to the physician immediately so that she may choose an appropriate treatment. Several classes of medication have been studied and have shown to be effective treatments for EPS, including anticholinergic medications, antihistamines, and benzodiazepines (Sharma et al., 2005). Not every class is equally effective for all types of EPS. The prescriber may try reducing the dosage or changing the antipsychotic medication in order to eliminate any EPS (Stanilla & Simpson, 2009).

It is not always easy to differentiate medication side effects from psychiatric symptoms. That is, it can be hard to differentiate akasthisia from anxiety and agitation, or a dystonic reaction from a psychotic posturing (Sharma, 2005). However, it is important that the treatment team attempt to do so because treatment for each may be different. The nurse should note whether there was any symptom relief shortly after administering a medication such as an anticholinergic medication or a benzodiazepine and communicate this to the prescriber so she can plan for continued treatment.

Serious adverse reactions. Less common but extremely serious reactions include neuroleptic malignant syndrome (NMS), serotonin syndrome, and lithium toxicity. These are potentially life threatening and require immediate medical attention. There is a great deal of information available in common drug references on these three significant adverse effects. It is imperative that nurses dispensing psychotropic medications become familiar with common signs and symptoms of these adverse reactions. Common indicators for these and other serious adverse reactions may include nausea and vomiting, diarrhea, fever, muscular rigidity, rapid change in blood pressure, and neuromuscular signs such as ataxia, tremulousness, and loss of coordination (Lee, 2010). These symptoms may occur quickly and require rapid attention by the nursing and medical staff. If a nurse suspects that the patient has symptoms of one of these conditions, he should hold the medication and contact the physician immediately.

DECISION MAKING

Holding a medication. The administration of medication is an area with a high potential for error. Many organizations and agencies focus risk management activities and quality initiatives on the reduction in medication errors. A nurse should hold a medication if he believes it may be causing a problem. Evidence of such problems may be found in the vital signs (including temperature reading, as this may indicate NMS), lab values, toxicity screens, or patient complaints. However, it is important to discuss the withholding of medications with the treating physician and seek guidance. There may be circumstances when the physician is aware of a problem but decides to go forward with treatment. For some medications, such as lithium or valproic acid, the acceptable therapeutic range differs depending on the reason for the treatment and the acceptable range may be higher than a lab's standard for that medication. For example, the therapeutic range for valproic acid is usually 50 to 100µg/ml. However, some prescribers may want the patient to have a level closer to 125µg/ml in cases of acute mania as long as there are no adverse effects (Schatzberg, Cole, & DeBattista, 2010).

The nurse is a valuable resource to the physician, in that she can watch carefully for adverse effects as well as help monitor lab values.

Increasing acceptance of medication. Sometimes a patient refuses medication, perhaps because he is psychotic and believes the medication to be poison, he dislikes the side effects, or he does not believe he needs the medication. Allowing the patient to have as much control as possible (within prescribing guidelines) may increase acceptance. For example, the patient may be able to choose the time of the medication ("now or 10 minutes from now"), the route ("liquid or pill form"), or the type of liquid ("water or apple juice"). Having a choice may engage the patient in the process enough that adherence increases. Coercion (such as saying, "If you don't take this medication, you will lose privileges," or linking avoidance of seclusion to the acceptance of a medication) is not acceptable; however, discussing the pros and cons of the medication with the patient may prove helpful. In some cases, certain medications (e.g., a cardiac medication or an antipsychotic medication) are most likely more important than other medications (e.g., a vitamin or a stool softener). If a patient is resistant to taking any medications, the nurse may negotiate with the patient to take the critical medication instead of the less important medication. Note that getting into struggles over acceptance of medication can lead to complications, such as an aggressive reaction from the patient. The nurse should consider the value of the medication, the desired effects, and the consequence if the medicine is not taken before getting into this struggle with the patient. As always, the nurse will discuss patient responses and concerns with the treatment team and prescriber.

Giving medication against a patient's will. Psychotropic medication can only be given against a patient's will in a case of specific and impending emergency (and only with a doctor's order), or with a court order for specific medication. Forcing a patient to take a medication is the last resort. The nurse should consult with other staff members, supervisors, and prescribers, if possible, before creating a potentially violent situation. The nurse must ensure that she has the legal right to administer the medication against the patient's will and have an adequate number of staff available. If she must force a medication on a patient, she should make contact with the patient after the event to reestablish the therapeutic alliance and allow the patient to debrief. The nurse can apologize for the event (but not the medication), review the reason for the medication, ask for the patient response to the medication, and work out a plan for the future. When a decision is made to give or not give a medication, the rationale should be clearly documented so that the treatment team is able to consider changing the treatment plan.

The prn medication. Medication is often ordered *pro re nata* or "as needed," and yet the evidence in the literature to the effectiveness of prn psychotropic medication is inconclusive (Baker, Lovell, & Harris, 2008; Shoumitro & Gemma, 2007; Usher, 2001; Usher, Baker, Holmes, Stocks, 2009). The physician order for a prn medication should spell out the actual reason it might be needed (e.g., headache) although sometimes the reason given is vague (agitation or anxiety). The utilization of psychotropic "prn" medication is a decision left to the medicating nurse (Usher, 2001). When deciding to administer a prn medication, the nurse should consider the following:

- Who is requesting the medication? Is it the patient, family members, or another staff person?
- Why is the medication requested or needed? What is the desired effect? Will it treat the symptom that the patient is complaining of or that the nurse observes?
- What other medications have already been given? What medications are yet to be given? What are the actions and side effects of all of the medications given? Are there any possible interactions among the medications and the prn?

If the patient requests the medication, the nurse will need to consider whether she agrees or believes the patient "needs" the medication. This is often an issue with pain or anxiety medications (see Chapters 6 and 2 respectively). Understanding the patient's goal for treatment, the physician's purpose for ordering the medication, and the expected outcome will help the nurse determine a course of action. However, if a physician orders the medication, there are no contraindications for giving the medication, and the time frame is not prohibited, then the nurse should give a prn if requested by the patient and discuss any lingering concerns with the treatment team.

If the nurse believes the patient needs a prn, he should still consider the questions outlined above as part of the decision-making process. The nurse should suggest the prn medication to the patient, discuss why it may be helpful, and discuss its desired effect.

Once a prn medication is given, the results should be evaluated within the hour. The nurse should document the patient response to the medication and communicate it to the treatment team and the physician. The nurse should also discuss alternatives to medication with the patient whether or not the medication has been given. Depending on the situation, this may include relaxation exercises, distraction, heat, or sensory interventions. These alternatives can sometimes be used instead of or in addition to the medication.

PATIENT MEDICATION EDUCATION

Medication education plays an important role in long-term adherence to the medication regime (Kemppainen et al., 2003). Adherence is different from compliance and implies the patient is an active participant in his care. Nurses have a responsibility to talk to patients about their medications and to provide information that clarifies and complements the information that the patient has from the pharmacy or physician. Engaging the patient in discussions around the medication prescribed allows the nurse not only to assess the willingness of the patient to take the medication, but also to include the patient actively in the process. This may increase the possibility that the patient will adhere to the treatment plan over time. The goal is to help the patient find a treatment regime that he will adhere to upon discharge. To that end, the patient's feelings, preferences, and experiences regarding medications are crucial information to be shared with the treatment team.

Any information given should be understandable, practical, unbiased, accurate, and presented in a manner that meets the individual needs of the patient. For example, the nurse may consider the patient's cognitive abilities and the level of privacy needed when deciding what to say about medication and how to say it. It is helpful to ask the patient's physician how much she has told the patient about the medication and request guidance in determining the level of education desired.

Medication education occurs in many forms, including individually at the time of administration, during one-to-one contact, and sometimes in a group (Morgan & Shoemaker, 2010). During medication administration, the nurse should always ask the patient if he knows what the medication is for and remind the patient of the name of the medication and the dosage. This prepares the patient for self-administration of medication in the future. During one-to-one contact, the nurse should invite the patient to ask questions, to discuss how he feels about taking this medication, and to talk about the experiences he has had with the medication to date. The nurse can then address any confusion or fear about the medication and review resources such as online medication information or printed patient education materials. In a group, the discussion about medications will be more general in order to provide information that will be useful for all the members. Potential group topics include

- Problem-solving about how to take medication in different circumstances (e.g., when at work)
- Interactions with alcohol and limitations on driving or other activities
- Types of medications
- Overall actions of medications
- Common side effects and strategies for coping with them

- General information about generic versus name brand medications
- Places to get additional information about medications
- Importance of talking with a physician or pharmacist for further information

Different agencies might have specific resources to be used for medication groups and the nurse should be familiar with these.

REFERENCES

Baker, J., Lovell, K., & Harris, N. (2008). A best-evidence synthesis review of the administration of psychotropic pro re nata (prn) medicaton in in-patient mental health settings. *Journal of Clinical Nursing, 17,*(9), 1122–1131.

Howland, R. (2011). Drug therapies for tardive dyskinesia. *Journal of Psychosocial Nursing, 48*(6), 13–20.

Janda, S., & Fagan, N. (2010). Practical review of pharmacology concepts. *Urologic Nursing, 30*(1), 15–21.

Kamin, J., Manwani, S., & Hughes, D. (2000). Extra pyramidal side effects in psychiatric emergency service. *Emergency Psychiatry, 51*(3), 288–289.

Kemppainen, J., Buffum, M., Wike, G., Kestner, M., Zappe, C., & Hopkins, R.,...Bartlebaugh, P. (2003). Psychiatric nursing and medication adherence. *Journal of Psychosocial Nursing and Mental Health, 41*(2), 38–49.

Lee, D. T. (2010). *Lithium toxicity clinical presentation.* Retrieved May 20, 2011, from http://emedicine.medscape.com/article/815523-clinical

Morgan, K., & Shoemaker, N. (2010). Therapeutic groups. In E. Varcarolis (Ed.), *Foundations of psychiatric mental health nursing* (pp. 742). St. Louis, MO: Saunders.

Schatzberg, A. F., Cole, J. O., & DeBattista, C. (2010). Mood stabilizers. In *Manual of clinical psychopharmacology* (7th ed.). Arlington, VA: American Psychiatric Publishing. doi: 10.1176/appi.books.9781585624119.604374

Sharma, A., Madaan,V., & Petty, F. (2005). Propranolol treatment for neuroleptic-induced akasthisia. *Primary Care Companion Journal of Clinical Psychiatry, 7*(4), 202–203.

Sherrod, R., Collins, A., Wynn S., & Gragg, M. (2010). Dissecting dementia, depression and drug effects in older adults. *Journal of Psychosocial Nursing, 48*(1), 39–47.

Shoumitro, D. & Gemma, L. U. (2007). Psychotropic medication for behaviour problems in people with intellectual disability: A review of the current literature. *Current Opinion Psychiatry, 20*(5), 461–466.

Stahl, S. M. (2000). *Essential psychopharmacology: Neuroscientific basis and practical applications* (2nd ed.). New York: Cambridge University Press.

Stanilla, J. K., & Simpson, G. M. (2009). Drugs to treat extra pyramidal side effects. In A. Schatzberg, & C. Nemeroff (Eds.), *American psychiatric publishing textbook of psychopharmacology* (4th ed.). Arlington, VA: American Psychiatric Publishing. doi: 10.1176/appi.books.9781585623860.430901

Usher, K., Baker, J. A., Holmes, C., & Stocks, B. (2009). Clincial decisionmaking for 'as needed' medications in mental health care. *Journal of Advanced Nursing, 65*(5), 981–991.

Usher, K. L. (2001). Mental health nurses' prn psychotropic medication administration. *Journal of Psychiatric Mental Health Nursing, 8*(5), 883–890.

World Health Organization, Collaborating Centre for Patient Safety Solutions. (2007). *Patient idenification.* Geneva, Switzerland: Author. Available at www.ccforpatientsafety.org/common/pdfs/pdf/presskit/PS-Solution2.pdf

Relaxation Techniques 13

Judy L. Sheehan

INTRODUCTION

Stress reduction and relaxation techniques, including diaphragmatic breathing, progressive muscle relaxation (PMR), and guided imagery and visualization are non-pharmacological nursing interventions that are frequently utilized on inpatient psychiatric units. Relaxation techniques can be used with many types of patients, and once a patient has learned a technique, it can be used in the hospital as frequently as the patient desires and also repeated at home. Because relaxation has been demonstrated to reduce insomnia, aggression, and anxiety, the implications for its use are broad (DeMarco-Sinatra, 2000). Relaxation training has been found to calm an overactive nervous system by reversing the negative effects of adrenalin on the body and reducing heart rate, respiratory rate, oxygen consumption, muscle tension, and blood pressure (DeMarco-Sinatra, 2000). Relaxation training may also increase active engagement in treatment and give the patient another healthy coping strategy to be used going forward. Relaxation training can take place in a group setting or with individual patients. The response patients have to this training should be communicated to the treatment teams and the nurses on the other shifts.

We present several simple relaxation techniques here. Choice of technique should largely be governed by patient preference.

DIAPHRAGMATIC BREATHING

Description. Shallow breathing can create increased feelings of anxiety and hyperventilation. The opposite of shallow breathing, that is, "diaphragmatic breathing" or "abdominal breathing," can be an effective mechanism for inducing relaxation. In this type of breathing, a person allows the lungs to slowly and completely fill with air using the abdominal muscles and thus relaxing the muscles that press against the diaphragm (McKay, Davis, & Fanning, 2007). The technique for teaching deep breathing is simple; the nurse instructs the patient to inhale to the count of four or five, pause and hold the breath to the count of five; and exhale to the count of five (DeMarco-Sinatra, 2000; Varcarolis and Halter, 2010; Kitko, 2007; Ross, 2008). Sometimes, it is useful to have the patient place her hand on her belly between the navel and the rib cage so that she can feel the rise of the abdomen as she breathes. If she is unable to breathe into her belly while sitting up (and instead only breathes shallowly, into her chest), the nurse can have the patient lie on her back with her hand on her belly and practice the technique.

This technique is most effective when a patient is able to focus on breathing in a quiet and comfortable environment. However, there are times when a patient may pace and become agitated, and it will be difficult for him to focus on the instructions or the breathing count. In these cases, the nurse can walk alongside the patient saying something like, "Breathe with me—it will help you relax." The nurse can then audibly breathe to the counts indicated above. There are times when just audibly breathing alongside a patient without saying anything will be sufficient.

When not to use. Some patients suffering with respiratory problems such as asthma or chronic obstructive pulmonary disease may find this activity difficult. If the patient begins to cough, complain of dizziness, or otherwise express discomfort, the nurse will have him cease the exercise, sit down, and resume normal breathing.

Resources. For more information, please see McKay et al. (2007), Olpin and Hesson (2007), and Smith (2002).

PROGRESSIVE MUSCLE RELAXATION

Description. PMR is one of the earliest forms of relaxation training and is sometimes called systematic muscle relaxation or Jacobson relaxation (DeMarco-Sinatra 2000; Vickers, Zollman & Payne, 2001). In this form of relaxation training, the patient is instructed to tense a group of muscles, hold the contraction for 10 or 15 seconds while breathing in, and release the tension while breathing out. The sequence is repeated in a systematic way, moving through all the major muscle groups. To teach this skill, the nurse can instruct the patient to start with the arms and tighten all muscles from the hands to the upper arms for 10 seconds, and then instruct the patient to allow the muscles to relax for about 20 seconds. Next, the nurse can have the patient tighten the muscles on his face by tightening or scrunching the brow, eyes, cheeks and lips for 10 seconds, then have him allow his face to relax for 20 seconds. The nurse will have the patient repeat the process with the torso muscles and then the leg and foot muscles. While doing this, the nurse should encourage the patient to notice the difference in sensation between tension and relaxation. The patient should be advised to tense the muscles in moderation and not to the point of discomfort. Note that the nurse will guide the patient through PMR rather than simply describe it to him and then leave him to do it. It is difficult to do this procedure without a guide unless one has had a lot of practice. There are also audio recordings available that will guide one through PMR. This process requires a quiet environment and may not be appropriate for all situations on an inpatient unit, but may be especially helpful for a patient having difficulty sleeping.

When not to use. A patient in pain or with physical limitations may not be able to participate in PMR. If a patient becomes uncomfortable or distressed during the process, she should be allowed to end the session.

Resources. For more information, please see McKay et al., (2007).

GUIDED IMAGERY AND VISUALIZATION

Description. Guided imagery and visualization allow for the induction of a relaxed state by having the patient induce a visual image that is pleasant and relaxing (McKay et al., 2007; Vickers, Zollman, & Payne, 2001). This may be a single image such as a flower or a tree, or a pleasant scene such as a beach or a forest. The image can be generated by the patient or offered by the nurse, but either way should be an image that the patient does not identify with trauma or negative emotion. The patient should be advised to close his eyes and focus on his breathing. After a moment or two, the patient should select a scene or natural item that he finds pleasant. He should be invited to stay with the image until he feels relaxed and then slowly open his eyes and bring his awareness back to the present situation. There are recorded guided relaxation sessions that can be utilized when available.

When not to use. This intervention may not be helpful for victims of trauma or abuse as it may trigger a flashback. The nurse should always monitor a patient undergoing guided imagery or visualization for indicators of anxiety or discomfort such as rapid breathing, distressed facial expressions, or hand or foot agitation. If the nurse notes distress, she should stop the session. For patients unable to tolerate guided visualization, other techniques such as deep breathing or PMR may be more appropriate.

Resources. Additional information can be found in McKay et al., (2007) or Olpin and Hesson (2007).

REFERENCES

DeMarco-Sinatra, J. (2000). Relaxation training as a holistic nursing intervention. *Holistic Nursing Practice, 14,* 30–39.

Kitko, J. (2007). Rhythmic breathing as a nursing intervention. *Holistic Nursing Practice, 21,* 85–88.

McKay, M., Davis, M., & Fanning, P. (2007). *Thoughts and feelings: Taking control of your mood and your life.* Oakland, CA: New Harbinger Publications.

Olpin, M., & Hesson, M. (2007). *Stress management for life: A research based experiential approach.* Belmont, CA: Thomson Company.

Ross, S. (2008). De-stressing the stress … naturally. *Holistic Nursing Practice, 22,* 365–368.

Smith, J. (2002). *Stress management: A comprehensive handbook of techniques and strategies.* New York: Springer Publishing.

Varcarolis, E., Halter, M., (2010). *Foundations of psychiatric mental health nursing.* St. Louis, MO: Saunders Elsevier.

Vickers, A. Z., Zollman, C., & Payne, D. K. (2001). Toolbox: Hypnosis and relaxation therapies. *Western Journal of Medicine, 175,* 269–272.

Sensory Interventions

Barbara Ostrove, Nancy Egan, and Susan Higgins

14

INTRODUCTION

The majority of people have the senses of sight, sound, touch, taste, and smell; yet, sensation is a subjective experience and helps to define uniqueness in personality and character. Understanding how each person perceives sensory information and how sensory information affects emotions allows nurses to help patients develop specific strategies to manage their illness.

In order to better understand the impact of the senses on emotions, the nurse might reflect on her own reactions. Consider the following questions:

- When you need to calm yourself, do you go for a run, lift weights, walk on the beach, listen to music, or take a shower with scented soap?
- What types of sensory input is distressing to you?
- Do you like walking around the mall during the holidays?
- Do you enjoy scented-candle shops or avoid them?
- Does the sand at the beach make you want to jump out of your skin?
- What sensory systems are involved in each of these activities?

The hospital environment can be one that is sensory sterile or sensory overloaded. Examples of what may make the environment sensory sterile include the following: patient bedrooms that are painted a muted color, group rooms that have no wall decorations, curtains that are often drawn shut on the windows, and furniture that is all the same institutional design. On the other hand, during meals, visiting hours, or at shift change, the unit can be very stimulating, with a lot of noise, movement, and smells. This environment does not always support optimal functioning in patients, in some cases can feel threatening or unpleasant, and can trigger behavioral outbursts (Champagne & Stromberg, 2004). Developing the ability to modulate one's response to sensations is an important component in learning to manage these situations (Champagne, 2008; Champagne & Stromberg, 2004).

Sensory modulation is defined as "the ability to organize and regulate one's reactions to sensory and motor stimulation in a graded and adaptive manner" (Bundy, Lane, & Murray as cited in Champagne, 2006b). Sensory interventions are the varied activities that are used to help with a sensory modulation program. They may be geared toward individuals or groups. The use of sensory interventions in mental health care provides a treatment option that can be tailored to each individual patient. Because the patient is taking an active role in his treatment, the use of these interventions can build self-esteem when the patient is successful. Patients with trauma histories may be particularly sensitive to sensation, so engaging in sensory interventions in a controlled way may allow them to normalize how they perceive sensation. The process of helping patients learn their sensory modulation preferences involves providing an environment that includes both active and passive activities from all areas of sensation. These sensory areas include not just sight, sound, taste, touch, and smell but also include vestibular sense (awareness of body position and the movement of the body) and proprioception (information from our joints and muscles that provides information on where one is in space).

There is a vast array of sensory interventions to put into a psychiatric nurse's therapeutic repertoire. Because of the diverse nature of the interventions, there is always something that can be used. Sensory activities can be either calming or alerting. An individualized balance of these activities can be thought of as a "sensory diet" (Wilbarger, 1995). Calming activities include those that are repetitive, are rhythmic, and involve deep pressure (i.e., proprioception). Foods that are sweet, are chewy, or can be sucked, and scents such as lavender or vanilla are usually calming. Activities that involve rapid change and movement such as running and kicking a ball, spicy foods, and sharp scents are all alerting. Although these are general rules, individuals can have unexpected reactions to certain activities or stimuli. For example, although lavender may be considered a calming scent, if it reminds a patient of a person with whom she had a traumatic experience, it may agitate her rather than calm her.

The remainder of this chapter will describe various types of sensory interventions that can be of benefit in a psychiatric treatment facility. They include sensory or comfort rooms, creating a comfortable milieu, sensory activities, sensory education groups, animal-assisted therapy (AAT), and the use of reduced sensory areas.

SENSORY OR COMFORT ROOMS

Description. Sensory rooms are specifically designated spaces designed to allow a patient to modulate his arousal and explore his sensory preferences (Champagne, 2006a). Most patients utilize these rooms to calm themselves, but in some cases, a patient may need to become *more* alert in order to fully engage in treatment. A sensory room can be used to increase alertness as well.

There is no standard for the development of sensory rooms, but they should always contain items from each area of sensation. The rooms should be developed in collaboration with staff and hospital leadership for every-one to understand their purpose. They are never to be used for seclusion, as this would give a patient a negative asso-ciation with the room, which will then negate the room's effectiveness in providing comfort. Smaller rooms are bet-ter than larger rooms. Locating the room in a quiet section of the unit is essential. It is important that these rooms have natural light and the opportunity to dim the lights. Finally, policies need to be designed to address infection control and safety concerns when patients are using the room.

Items to be included in a sensory room:

- Tactile: Stress balls, koosh balls, fabrics of varying tex-tures, worry stones, clay, and fidgets (e.g., hand puzzles, tangles, or a slinky)
- Visual: Picture books, relaxation DVDs, murals, lami-nated pictures of relaxing places, fish tanks, lava lamps, and glitter wands
- Auditory: Music and relaxation CDs, rain sticks, musical instruments, sound machines, headphones, and porta-ble music players
- Olfactory: Scented lotions, scented electric candles, cin-namon sticks, vanilla beans, lemons, and air fresheners.
- Gustatory: Lollipops, hard candy, red hot fire balls, sour patch candy, mints, sugar-free gum, and pretzels.
- Movement/deep pressure: Rocker/recliner, weighted blankets, Thera-Band, therapy balls, and vibrating massagers.

Note that many of these items fall into several sensory cat-egories. Scented lotions provide tactile and olfactory input, and environmental DVDs are both visual and auditory.

Nursing role. All patients can benefit from using the sensory room. The nurse should decide how much super-vision is needed for each patient and remember that patients will need assistance to understand the purpose of the room. It is essential to educate patients about the sensory room when they are being oriented to the unit. Having an awareness of the room as a resource allows patients to choose to use the room and empowers them to take responsibility for calming themselves. When needed, the nurse should cue patients that the room is available for use or provide them with supplies from the room if the room is occupied. The nurse may help the patients explore sensory activities and discuss with them the helpfulness of the selected activity and ways to incorporate these activities into their daily routines.

When not to use. Although the purpose of the sensory room is to help patients explore and understand their sensory preferences, it is often used to help patients de-escalate. Patients who are already agitated should not be referred to use the room because a sensory room may be overstimulating to these patients. These patients are at risk for injuring themselves or damaging supplies. Instead, the nurse should provide an agitated patient with a strategy to use in his room.

Resources. For more information, please see Champagne, T. (2006), Champagne, R. (2006), Champagne (2008), and Champagne and Stromberg (2004).

CREATING A COMFORTABLE MILIEU

Description. Although the use of sensory rooms is very effective, they are limited by the number of patients who can use the room at any given time. It is important to create a sensory-friendly unit that will help patients and visitors feel more comfortable throughout their time on the unit. This can be challenging as everyone may have different ideas about what would make a unit "comfortable." However, general guidelines would include having adequate seating, natural lighting, areas for quiet and stimulating activities, and areas that provide changes in sound, scents, and sights. Simple gestures such as turning down the overhead fluorescent lights or using battery-powered scented candles can change the mood and tone of the unit.

Nursing role. Along with constantly evaluating the patients on the unit, the nurse should be monitoring the sensory nature of the unit. Nursing staff should pay attention to all the senses. Is the unit getting too noisy? Or is it too quiet? What is the visual appearance? How does it smell? Nurses can encourage unit staff to take an active role in making changes to the environment to provide balance and to make it more comfortable. Nurses may also consider having a focus group discussion with patients to learn their thoughts about the unit and to allow the patients to provide suggestions on what would make the unit more comfortable.

SENSORY ACTIVITIES

Description. Sensory activities should be built into the course of the day on the unit. This will allow patients to understand and appreciate their effectiveness, so they will seek them out as needed. This also helps to create a pleasant and engaging treatment milieu.

Sensory activities can be effective with all patients. Patients with anxiety, trauma histories, borderline personality disorder, and mood disorders can often identify particular activities that may help manage their symptoms. Patients with psychotic disorders find these same activities organizing. Sensory activities can occur in a group setting or be an individual activity. Activities might include cooking, self-care activities (foot baths, hot stone massages, manicures, or pedicures), or craft activities. Craft activities can include making small pillows with an aromatherapy scent added to the inside or making soap and homemade skin care products. Even an activity like popping popcorn on the unit can be an aromatherapy activity that will draw people out of their rooms and encourage socialization.

Nursing role. Nurses generally play a supportive role in helping sensory activities happen. They can encourage staff to be creative when planning milieu activities, direct budgetary funds toward unit supplies, and provide education to physicians and administration. However, patients find great value in small gestures from nurses, such as providing warm milk when they are unable to sleep, supplying herbal tea, or providing scented hand lotion. These can all help nurses to build rapport with patients.

When not to use. As with all sensory strategies, the nurse should evaluate the patient before engaging her in an activity. In particular, the nurse should be careful with patients who are agitated. Handing supplies to a patient who is agitated may provide him with something to throw as opposed to using as intended.

SENSORY EDUCATION GROUP

Description. A sensory education group can be used to help patients learn different ways in which they may regulate their mood via sensory input. To lead this group, the nurse will need to have some objects from each sensory category available. A portable cart with items from the sensory room is ideal. The following is a sample group protocol for a sensory education group.

Introduction. First, the nurse will draw a table with six columns and three rows on a whiteboard. In the first column, in the middle cell, he can write "Calming" and in the last cell, he can write "Alerting." He may then say, "Today we are going to talk about our sensory systems. We have five senses, can you name them?" The nurse will fill in the five senses across the top of the chart on the whiteboard. Movement and deep pressure can be included as additional categories. He may go on to say, "We experience our world everyday through our senses, and so today we are going to discuss ways in which we can regulate ourselves in order to alert or calm our bodies. Sensory activities can provide ways to deal with symptoms such as anxiety, frustration, and agitation." He can then ask patients to identify activities that they find calming or alerting and fill in these activities in the appropriate boxes.

Activity. The group leader can then engage the group in a brief movement activity such as balloon volleyball, stretching, or a ball toss in order to demonstrate how movement can wake people up. Next, the group leader will introduce each of the five sensory categories one by one and allow group members a few minutes to experience the sensory supplies. Finally, the nurse can introduce deep-pressure activities as a way for patients to feel calmer. Although getting a massage or lifting weights is not possible in this setting, these activities can be simulated by using vibrating toys or stretching a Thera-Band. It is best to remove each set of supplies before introducing a new sensory category to minimize distraction.

Processing. Finally, the group leader or nurse will provide an opportunity for each participant to discuss their sensory likes and dislikes. He may ask a number of questions: "How did you feel about doing this activity? How did it feel to experience different sensory modalities? What did you learn about yourself by doing this activity? What activities were calming? What activities woke you up? How can you schedule sensory strategies into your weekly routine at home? Can you identify a situation or time of day where you could use one of your sensory preferences to calm or alert yourself? How can you use these strategies to help you during your treatment?"

When not to use. Patients should always be evaluated before being included in groups. If a patient is very manic or agitated, they may not be able to tolerate the group. This group can be adapted to have less discussion and primarily focus on sensory exploration; this may be more effective with patients with lower cognitive functioning.

ANIMAL-ASSISTED ACTIVITIES AND AAT

Description. In mental health facilities, providing dogs in the milieu can have numerous benefits. Having dogs in the milieu can lower blood pressure, decrease stress, and increase social interactions. Dogs help provide a sense of psychological and emotional wellness, which in turn may help patients overcome feelings of depression and loneliness. Finally, dogs can provide a sense of safety, support, and trust, which is often missing in the mental health milieu (Brown, 2009).

Dogs can be used with all ages. With children and adolescents, dogs help demonstrate basic obedience, teach calming strategies, and stimulate play. On the adult units, the use of dogs in the therapeutic milieu promotes socialization, reduces feelings of isolation and depression, and encourages positive feelings. On the geriatric unit, the dogs can help patients improve memory and organization while providing sensory experiences through touch, sight, sound, and deep pressure (Brown, 2009).

Most dogs in mental health facilities are used for animal-assisted activities (AAA). AAA "provide opportunities for motivation, education, or recreation to enhance quality of life. Animal assisted activities are delivered in a variety of environments by specially trained professionals, paraprofessionals, or volunteers in association with animals that meet specific criteria" (http://www.avma. org/issues/policy/animal_assisted_guidelines.asp). AAA includes regularly scheduled "meet and greets," where the dogs spend time with patients on the units, demonstrating tricks, sitting to be petted, or just making contact with individuals. During these times, many patients who generally spend time in their rooms may come out into the open areas just to pet the dogs and watch what is going on. These times also provide structure to the day and introduce something "new" to the normal hospital routine.

AAA can be contrasted with Animal-assisted therapy (AAT), which is "a goal directed intervention in which an animal meeting specific criteria is an integral part of the treatment process. Animal-assisted therapy is delivered and/or directed by health or human service providers working within the scope of their profession. Animal-assisted therapy is designed to promote improvement in human physical, social, emotional, or cognitive function. Animal-assisted therapy is provided in a variety of settings, and may be group or individual in nature. The process is documented and evaluated" (http://www.avma.org/issues/policy/animal_assisted_guidelines.asp).

Thus, AAT is the goal-directed use of dogs for a therapeutic outcome. In these instances, dogs are included in the treatment plan as a nontraditional method for achieving behavioral outcomes. For example, the patient who is too psychotic to go to groups can be involved in one-to-one sessions with the dog to "teach" the dog tricks and basic obedience commands. As the patient becomes comfortable talking with the dog, she may then feel more comfortable talking to her treatment team and peers on the unit.

Nursing role. Nurses are a vital part of facilitating positive animal-assisted interactions. Nurses are aware of the status of individual patients and communicate this information to the animal handler. Nurses can also relay information to the handler as to which patients may benefit from AAA/AAT and which patients should not be involved due to infection, physical limitations, or behavioral status. Nurses can also evaluate and communicate the effectiveness of the AAA/AAT intervention to the treatment team.

During AAA/AAT, nurses can assist by watching for signs of stress in the patients and the animals. Patients who are stressed may react violently or may become confused and disoriented, causing harm to patients and therapy pets. Therapy pets used in AAA/AAT that are stressed may also become defensive, trying to get away from the uncomfortable situation, and harming patients in their way. If a nurse notices signs of stress, she can act immediately to avoid a potentially dangerous situation.

When not to use AAA/AAT. AAA/AAT is not beneficial for people who have a fear of animals and especially people who have been diagnosed with posttraumatic stress disorder, anxiety disorders, or obsessive–compulsive disorder related to animals. AAA/AAT should not be used with people who have an allergy to animals. Finally, for the safety of both the therapy pet and the patient, therapy pets should not be used with people with severe psychosis and unpredictable behaviors.

Resources for more information. For more information on implementing an AAA/AAT program, refer to the Delta Society (1999; www.deltasociety.org), or Therapy Dogs International (www.tdi-dog.org).

REDUCED SENSORY AREAS

Description. Therapeutic nursing interventions also include the consideration of other areas that offer less stimulation (i.e., less noise, less contact with peers) than comfort rooms or sensory rooms. The open-door quiet room is an option that is available for the patient who seeks less stimulation than the above-mentioned rooms and is not his assigned sleeping area.

Patients who are seeking a space to have less stimulation may request to use the quiet room or it may be offered to them. The benefits can include an opportunity for the patient to feel safe, to ask for what she needs, and to take responsibility in self-modulation or self-calming by controlling her own environment (Champagne, 2006b). The patient who requests the quiet room may have been traumatized as a child or as an adult and perceive the world around her as a potential threat. Use of the quiet room or other quiet space may be a means to control her responses to anticipated harm (Ziegler, 2003).

Guidelines for use of the open-door quiet room:

- Placing the patient on frequent checks
- Keeping the door open and in a locked position to prevent inadvertent or purposeful closing
- Allowing the patient egress at any time.

Sensory items may be provided when requested, although if the patient asks for them or the staff offers them and they are accepted, staff should also offer a transition to the bedroom or sensory room.

The open-door quiet room may also serve as a space that is suitable for the patient who has been in the locked-door quiet room, providing him with a transition area before rejoining the milieu. For this patient, the length of time spent there is determined by both patient self-assessment and staff assessment. The staff assessment may include vital signs and a preliminary patient debriefing. The debriefing is an essential procedure when terminating seclusion. The preliminary debriefing is an assessment of patient affect and physical well-being. The complete debriefing may take place over hours and sometimes days, and includes reviewing facts related to an event in addition to processing the response to them. It provides the patient and staff with an opportunity to clarify the rationale for seclusion, offer mutual feedback, and identify alternative methods of coping that might help the patient avoid seclusion in the future.

Nursing role. Ideally, the decision to use the open-door quiet room will be a collaborative one between the nurse and the patient. The nurse and patient should discuss the goals and benefits of its use, with a focus on the patient's strengths and resiliency. The patient may have insight from previous experience in which the quiet room was a good tool for assisting her with coping with stress and helping her to regain a previous state of control and normalcy.

Before using the quiet room, the nurse should explore alternative self-calming strategies with the patient. These may be strategies that the patient has not tried in the past or strategies she has not thought about using in the current environment. This process of exploring alternatives may meet several patient needs. One-to-one time with a caring staff may provide a perception of safety. When this conversation occurs in a quiet, peaceful part of the unit, there is a decrease in other environmental stimulation. The nurse may suggest that the patient consider writing, listening to music, taking a warm shower, doing relaxation exercises, or engaging in other quiet activities that may satisfy the patient's need for decreased stress. The nurse and patient may decide that these strategies be tried in addition to or instead of the open-door quiet room.

When not to use the open-door quiet room. This room should not be used when the patient is unusually anxious or is reacting in other ways that are suggestive of re-experiencing trauma. The patient who wants to hide and is extremely anxious will need to be observed closely in the milieu or in another more visible area, such as his bedroom. The best practice is to have input from the treatment team to guide clinical decisions regarding quiet room use with any patients who are dissociating, psychotic, or socially isolative.

REFERENCES

Brown, D. P. (2009) *Animal assisted therapy: The layman's guide to animal assisted therapy*. Retrieved from http://learninglifeebooks.com

Champagne, T. (2006a). Creating sensory rooms: Environmental enhancements for acute inpatient mental health settings. *Mental Health Special Interest Section Quarterly, 29*(4), 1–4.

Champagne, T. (2006b). *Sensory modulation and environment: Essential elements of occupation* (2nd ed.). Southampton, MA: Champagne Conferences and Consultation.

Champagne, T. (2008). Sensory modulation program for adolescents & adults. Retrieved December 15, 2008, from http://www.ot-innovations.com

Champagne, T., & Stromberg, N. (2004). Sensory approaches in inpatient psychiatric settings. *Journal of Psychosocial Nursing, 42*(9), 1–8.

Delta Society. (1999). *Standards of practice for animal-assisted activities and therapy*. Renton, WA: Author.

Wilbarger, P. (1995). The sensory diet: Activity programs based upon sensory processing theory. *Sensory Integration Special Interest Section Quarterly, 18*(2), 1–4.

Ziegler, D. (2003). *Traumatic experience and the brain: A handbook for understanding and treating those traumatized as children*. Phoenix, AZ: Acacia Publishing Inc.

Therapeutic One to One

Laura Drury, Diane Ferreira,
Joanne M. Matthew, and Lisa A. Uebelacker

15

INTRODUCTION

The therapeutic nurse–patient relationship is the corner-stone of psychiatric nursing practice. Numerous studies across mental health professions have found that a positive therapeutic relationship between the patient and caregiver is associated with positive treatment outcomes (Dziopa & Ahern, 2009). A review of evidence-based nursing litera-ture yields common interpersonal attributes of the nurse that contribute to a quality nurse–patient relationship. These include being genuine, providing empathy and understanding, maintaining clear boundaries, and regular patient contact (Scanlon, 2006). The therapeutic one-to-one interaction is a very important opportunity for the nurse to build a positive relationship with his patients.

The overarching goal of therapeutic one-to-one con-tact is to help the patient move toward achieving optimal health. The nurse may use this time to conduct assess-ment, make efforts to engage the patient, or provide vari-ous interventions. The nurse can briefly touch on each of these three types of goals (i.e., assessment, engagement, or intervention) or focus on a single category, depending on the patient's condition and the time allotted for the contact.

ELEMENTS OF THE ONE-TO-ONE CONTACT

Assessment

There are many aspects of the patient's experience that can be assessed during the one-to-one contact. The nurse may assess

- Behavior, including his body language, rate and volume of speech, and degree of eye contact
- Ability to concentrate on the conversation
- Orientation to his/her surroundings, including date, time, and place
- Personal hygiene
- Symptoms, including the patient's mood, safety, thought processes, sleep, appetite, and other symptoms that are treatment targets, which is done through direct questioning
- Comorbid medical and psychiatric symptoms
- Perception of treatment and its effectiveness. The nurse asks questions about the perceived effectiveness of medications and how the patient feels about his hospital stay
- Potential side effects from psychiatric medications. The nurse can directly ask the patient if she thinks she is having any side effects. Alternatively, the nurse can ask about symptoms reflective of side effects, such as feeling tired or dizzy, having trouble with urination, or constipation. The nurse also looks for possible behavioral manifestations of side effects, such as somnolence, agitation, or delirium (Huggins, 2006).
- Behaviors and reactions that may be influenced by the patient's culture and ethnicity

Note that the nurse will need to decide which of these aspects of the patient experience are most important to assess in a given contact. He will likely not assess everything at every contact.

Engagement

Promoting and encouraging the patient's engagement in treatment is another crucial aspect of therapeutic one-to-one contact.

Beginning the contact. From the first moment, when the nurse meets the patient, she begins to build the foundation of the therapeutic relationship. The nurse introduces herself and explains her role on the treatment team. She also attends to the patient's immediate concerns for comfort and safety, as well as answers questions (Deering & Mohr, 2006). The nurse may use the following open-ended questions to encourage the patient to open up:

- Could you tell me in your own words what has brought you to the hospital?
- How are you feeling today?
- How has your stay been so far?
- What are you most concerned about?

Listening. Attentive listening is crucial to building the nurse–patient relationship. By the nurse attentively listening, the patient comes to feel understood, and the nurse gains an understanding of the patient's needs. Attentive listening is a skill that involves being fully present and hearing and conveying understanding of what the patient is saying, as well as what is not being said (Forchuk & Boyd, 2005).

Examples of how the nurse listens attentively include

- Making good eye contact
- Addressing the patient by his proper name
- Being available and fully present with the patient
- Being curious about the patient's experience. For example, the nurse may say, "Could you help me to understand what you mean by that?" or "What is the most difficult part of this for you?"

- Asking open-ended questions
- Reflecting and summarizing what the patient has said. For example, the nurse might say, "You've said that you feel hopeless and fearful about the future. Have I got that right?"
- Taking care not to pass judgment, and to make an effort to show acceptance of the patient's experience
- Remembering that silence can be soothing to the distressed patient

Nursing behaviors that could decrease treatment engagement. There are also ways in which the nurse could unintentionally diminish the patient's sense of self and desire to engage in treatment. Therefore, the nurse should consider the following guidelines:

- Address the patient by her proper name; do not use other terms such as "honey" or "sweetie."
- In general, do not touch patients. There is a debate by nursing scholars about the therapeutic use of touch with psychiatric patients. Nursing research has found that physical touch (i.e., holding a patient's hand, placing a hand on the patient's hand, or hugging a patient) can be comforting to many patients, but other patients can become distressed when touched (Routasalo, 1999). For example, patients suffering from psychosis can become agitated or violent when touched; those who have experienced physical abuse can panic when touched. Patients whose culture has prohibitions against being touched may feel violated. Therefore, it is wise to express warmth and caring through kind words of encouragement and refrain from using touch as a mechanism for reassurance and comfort.
- Refrain from premature or unrealistic reassurance. Well-intended statements like "Don't worry; it will be fine" can result in the patient feeling her concerns are being minimized.

- Do not give advice or personal opinion. Statements like "I'd tell him to leave; you don't deserve to be treated like that," or "Don't let her upset you" may be intended to reassure and support the patient. Such statements can be infantilizing, however, and can cause the patient to feel criticized and cause her not to communicate further. Instead, the nurse should encourage the patient to explore her own feelings and develop effective coping skills. In this way, the nurse helps the patient to develop self-understanding and increase a sense of hope that they can effect important changes.
- Use self-disclosure sparingly. When the nurse shares his own experiences, this takes the focus away from the patient. A good question to ask oneself before making a disclosure is, "Would I be sharing this if my supervisor were here?" Instead of using self-disclosure, the nurse should be curious about the patient's unique experience. He can ask questions to help the patient explore what she is feeling and what she thinks would be helpful.
- Do not take the patient's anger or negative expressions personally. It is helpful for the nurse who finds herself to be the recipient of a patient's hostility to remember that most likely the patient is frightened and distressed.
- Do not deceive or manipulate the patient. The nurse–patient relationship is built on trust.
- Be careful when using humor. The nurse should take her cue from the patient in determining his comfort level with humor. The nurse should never tease a psychotic patient or another patient who may not understand the subtext.

Managing patient expectations. Patients often have expectations that cannot be met, for example, about what kind of communication they will have with the nurse, how often communication will occur, and how the nurse can meet their needs. The nurse must manage this in a way that promotes patient engagement and trust, while still setting some boundaries with the patient. In these cases, the nurse should thoughtfully educate the patient and explain why the expectation cannot be met. Often the patient will find this helpful. The nurse can also offer an alternative that may help meet patient needs but that stays within the boundaries of what the nurse is able to offer.

In particular, some patients will want more contact time than the nurse is able to give. For example, the patient who is overwhelmed with anxiety might say, "I can't take it any more, please don't leave. I need you to stay with me." In this case, the nurse will be aware of the patient's desperation and sense of hopelessness. In response, the nurse might say, "John, I'll stay with you for a while, but then I will have to pass medications. But I will check in with you periodically to see how you are doing." In this case, frequent but brief supportive contact may help the patient feel heard and cared about. In addition, the nurse can help the patient identify some stress-reducing techniques and encourage the patient to practice these techniques between meeting times with the nurse.

Intervention

The last goal for the one-to-one contact is to provide an intervention. The nurse helps the patient to identify goals, develop effective means of coping or stress-reduction techniques, and problem solve. The nurse also provides education and information about medications and treatments. This part of the one to one should be tailored to individual needs of the patient, but any patient can benefit from information about her condition, medications, relapse prevention, or discharge plans.

Help the patient to identify goals or more effective means of coping with her illness. Suggested questions include

- What would you like to be different about your situation?

- If you make changes, how would your life be different?
- What will happen if you don't change?
- What has been of help to you in the past?
- How can I help you get past some of these difficulties?

(Miller and Rollnick, 2002)

In this discussion, the nurse may gently challenge a patient to look at things differently or consider making changes in his life. It is possible that the patient will experience this as minimizing his difficulties. If so, the nurse explains that her intention is to assist the patient in recognizing his ability to effect important changes. In this way, the nurse fosters a sense of hope by sharing her belief that the patient can better his life.

For example, the nurse may say, "Fred, I can see that you're upset that I'm asking you to look at things differently, but please understand that I mean to be of help to you. I'm concerned for your health and your marriage. If you continue drinking, what do you think will happen?" As another example, the nurse may say, "Joan, I know you're irritated that I'm giving you a bit of a push. Please know that it's coming from a sense of caring. So please think about attending the family meeting. You'll be leaving before you know it and this is your opportunity, with support, to work things out."

Help the patient problem solve. Key elements of problem solving include problem identification, brainstorming about different possible solutions without judging them, exploring the pros and cons of each solution, choosing a solution to try, and then evaluating how well the solution worked. The nurse can help the patient to problem solve with some of the following questions:

- What, exactly, is the problem? Why is it a problem?
- What are possible solutions to this problem? Let's brainstorm. That means, let's think of lots of different

possibilities, no matter how unlikely they seem. After we do this, we'll look at which solution seems best.

- What are the pros and cons of this solution? What will it mean for you or your family in the short term? In the long term?
- Given our discussion, what would you like to try first?

Help the patient identify stress-reduction techniques. The nurse can help the patient identify some stress-reducing techniques and encourage the patient to practice these techniques between meeting times with the nurse. By remembering to talk with the patient regarding how he was able to utilize the new coping strategies, the nurse demonstrates that she cares about the patient's progress. If the patient has not been able to practice the stress-reducing techniques, the nurse can help the patient to identify barriers and offer brief support to the patient. For the patient who was able to utilize the stress-reducing techniques successfully, the nurse gives the patient positive feedback to reinforce the new learned behavior.

Provide the patient with information about medications and treatments such as electroconvulsive therapy. Please see Chapter 12, "Medication Administration," for more detailed information about providing medication education. Complete education about treatments can be given over the course of several sessions. The elements of education needed for medication and for electroconvulsive therapy are similar. In brief, education will include the following: name, purpose, and dose of medication (or other treatment); common side effects, including how long they will last; any symptoms that should be reported immediately to the nurse; and necessary lab tests that may accompany the treatment. The nurse should also carefully answer any patient questions.

There are a few other guidelines that the nurse can keep in mind. The nurse will repeat and further explain any education provided by the prescriber. Repetition is useful for many patients. The nurse should tailor the education to the cognitive abilities of the patient. Finally, it is often helpful to provide written or visual education materials in addition to verbal instructions.

Ending the Session

As the session comes to an end, the nurse will ask the patient how he is feeling and what he thought of the session. If the patient states that the session was helpful, the nurse can inquire, "What was helpful?" or "What will you take away from the session?" If the patient says, the session was upsetting or not helpful, the nurse can ask, "Can you help me understand what was upsetting about our session? What would have been more helpful?" Having the opportunity to address and correct any misunderstanding, distortions, or negative feelings should strengthen the alliance between the nurse and patient.

Next, the nurse should summarize the session by restating both the content and feelings expressed by the patient. She can also remind the patient that staff are available for help on every shift. A closing statement that is positive can give the patient encouragement to get through the day or evening. Finally, the nurse should let the patient know when they will meet again.

An example of a summary of a one-to-one session initiated by the nurse is: "Susan, we need to end our time together for today. You've shared some very private and painful things this afternoon; thank you for making the effort to share them with me. Being diagnosed with breast cancer is devastating. And I can hear your ambivalence—you want to protect your family from worrying by not telling them, and yet you also need their support. You've been under tremendous stress. So, I'm glad you've agreed to start an antidepressant. Please remember that the staff is here for you. Let's plan to meet tomorrow at the same time. Any questions? … Have a good night, and I'll see you tomorrow." If the contact was initiated by the patient, then the nurse might say, "I hope that I was able to answer your question" and go on to explain what steps he will take as a result of the meeting.

FREQUENCY AND LENGTH OF ONE-TO-ONE CONTACT

A key issue for nurses is the numerous and sometimes conflicting responsibilities that limit the time they have to spend with their patients. Although this is a real tension, whenever possible it is best to sit down with each patient, even for a short while, in a quiet and private area on the inpatient unit. While nurses meet with their patients once per waking shift, for patients who are highly anxious and require more reassurance, it is helpful to have a shorter and more frequent contact. The nurse should also let the patient know when he will meet with the patient again; this is reassuring to the patient. The nurse should be certain to follow through with any commitment he has made to the patient. If the nurse is unable to keep a commitment to meet with the patient, he should offer another time to meet.

Therapeutic contact can be brief. The nurse can demonstrate caring even when he only has a brief contact. The nurse can make statements that convey awareness of the patient's day-to-day progress and also show that he remembers what is important to the patient (e.g., names of family members, personal situations). For example, the nurse might say, "John, I notice that you've been on the unit more today, it's nice to see you spending time out of your room. I saw that your granddaughter, Lily, visited you earlier today." Another example is: "Mary, were you able to reach Bob last night? I know you were concerned about how he made out on his first day of student teaching." This conveys to the patient that he is important and the nurse cares about his progress.

CULTURE AND ETHNICITY

Everyone has a cultural and ethnic heritage that contributes to a person's sense of self and how he interacts with his environment. Moreover, beliefs about illness and mental health are greatly influenced by a person's culture and ethnicity. For many patients, religion is a source of strength and comfort. It is important for the nurse to be aware of and examine his own beliefs, as well as any cultural stereotypes, biases, and prejudices. In addition to cultural and ethnic differences, the nurse also needs to be aware of subcultures such as gay, lesbian, bisexual, and transgender groups, and the homeless. The nurse who has an understanding of different cultures will be better able to provide care that is in concert with the patient's beliefs and background (Boyd, 2005).

For example, the nurse who has an understanding of Chinese culture will be mindful that a Chinese patient who does not make eye contact may do so in deference to the nurse's authority. A Haitian woman who is praying the Rosary and reading a prayer book daily may be mistaken by staff as being hyperreligious when in fact she is engaging in a common cultural practice. An Ethiopian man who is being treated for mania may have family who believe he is ill due to evil spirits; this is a common belief in the Ethiopian culture (Lipson, Dibble, & Minarik, 1998).

These are a few examples that illustrate the need for the nurse to continue professional development through ongoing education of diverse cultural norms and practices. This can be completed through formal continuing education or through informal reading or talking with members of a community. The nurse can also learn about cultural practices by carefully listening to patients and their families.

While a complete discussion of cultural, racial, and ethnic competencies is beyond the scope of this book, the following key points are important for the nurse to assess in the context of a one-to-one interaction:

- To what extent does the patient identify with their ethnic group?
- Could a patient's seemingly unusual behavior be normal within her cultural group?
- Does the patient have ethnic or religious practices that are important to them?
- What is the patient's sense of family? The nurse will allow the patient to define the composition of their family by asking the patient who is in her family.
- Does the patient have any ethnic or religious food preferences or restrictions?
- What is the patient's preference for language? The nurse should not assume that the patient who speaks English as a second language is able to fully comprehend what is being said. The nurse must be aware of the interpreter policies of his institution

McGoldrick, Pearce, & Giordano (1982).

The nurse will want to provide a unit atmosphere that encourages patients to express themselves through eating and food rituals, dress, sleep, and healing and care activities as long as it does not violate institutional policies.

REFERENCES

Boyd, M. (2005). Cultural issues related to mental health care. In M. Boyd (Ed.), *Psychiatric nursing, contemporary practice* (pp. 18–21). Philadelphia, PA: Lippincott, Williams & Wilkins.

Deering, C., & Mohr W. (2006).Therapeutic relationships and communication. In W. Mohr (Ed.), *Psychiatric mental health nursing* (pp. 56–61). Philadelphia, PA: Lippincott, Williams & Wilkins.

Dziopa, F., & Ahern, K. (2009). What makes a quality therapeutic relationship in psychiatric/mental health nursing: A review of the research. *The Internet Journal of Advanced Nursing Practice 10*(1). Retrieved August 22, 2011, from http://www.ispub.com/journal/the-internet-journal-of-advanced-nursing-practice/volume-10-number-1/what-makes-a-quality-therapeutic-relationship-in-psychiatric-mental-health-nursing-a-review-of-the-research-literature.html

Forchuk, F., & Boyd. A. (2005). Publication and the therapeutic relationship. In A. Boyd (Ed.), *Psychiatric nursing contemporary practice* (pp. 175–183). Philadelphia, PA: Lippincott, Williams & Wilkins.

Huggins, M. (2006). Culture. In W. Mohr (Ed.), *Psychiatric mental health nursing* (pp.81–84). Philadelphia, PA: Lippincott, Williams & Wilkins.

Lipson, J., Dibble, S., & Minarik, P. (1998). *Culture and nursing care.* San Francisco, CA: UCSF Nursing Press.

McGoldrick, M., Pearce, J., & Giordano, J. (1982). *Ethnicity and family therapy.* New York: Guilford Press.

Miller, W., & Rollnick, S. (2002). *Motivational interviewing: Preparing people for change* (2 ed.). New York: Guilford Press.

Routasalo, P. (1999). Physical touch in nursing studies: A literature review. *Journal of Advanced Nursing, 30,* 843–850.

Scanlon, A. (2006). Psychiatric nurse's perception of the constituents of the relationship: A grounded theory of study. *Journal of Psychiatric Nursing Mental Health Nursing, 13,* 319–329.

Managing Violence 16

Judy L. Sheehan

INTRODUCTION

Episodes of violence can be seen as having a beginning, a middle, and an end. The beginning is that time prior to the actual violence, when de-escalation and environmental management is essential. The middle of the episode is when the violence actually occurs, when the goal is to maintain safety and restore calm. The end occurs once the episode is over. In this chapter, we discuss essential elements of nursing intervention in each of these phases.

PREPARATION: BEFORE THE BEGINNING

Know safety procedures at one's own agency. It is important to have good understanding of the safety procedures for one's own agency. An organization's plan for dealing with psychiatric emergencies should reflect federal and state regulations and should include procedures for how to call for help, how to segregate aggressive persons from other patients and visitors, and what safety equipment is available and how to use it. (Safety equipment may include shields, face masks, stretchers, etc.) It is also important to know where exits, alarms, and emergency equipment are located in every unit in which one works. Nurses should be sure to be well acquainted with the psychiatric emergency safety plan for their agency.

BEGINNING: PREVENTION AND DE-ESCALATION

Be aware of indicators for impending violence. Violence may seem to erupt on an inpatient psychiatric unit quickly and unexpectedly. In many cases, indicators of impending violence may have been present, but because of the dynamics of the milieu, the staffing focus, or the scheduling of groups, the early indicators may not have been noticed by the staff. In order to promote a safe environment, it is helpful to anticipate potentially violent situations so that preventive measures can be initiated (Vaaler, 2011). Some of the indicators that a patient is becoming distressed and potentially aggressive may be an increased respiratory rate, clenched fists, and changes in facial color or expressions. The tone of voice may become louder and angrier, speech may become more rapid, and the patient may begin to pace or stare or glare at another patient or staff member. (For more information, please see Chapter 1, The Patient With Anger; Chapter 3, "The Patient With Disorganized Behavior," and Chapter 7, "The Patient With Paranoia").

A number of scales designed to predict violence are available and can be used by nursing staff on inpatient units. Examples of these include the Forensic Early Warning Signs of Aggression Inventory (Fluttert, Van Meijel, Van Leeuwen, Bjorkly, & Nijman, 2011), The Classification of Violence Risk (McDermott, 2011), The Broset Violence Checklist (Clarke & Griffith, 2010), and the Staff Observation Aggression Scale–Revised (Vaaler, 2011). These scales provide a systematic way in which nurses can be looking for early warning signs.

De-escalate. When a potentially dangerous situation has been identified, nurses and other staff must make attempts to "de-escalate" or "defuse" the situation. The first thing that the nurse will often do is try to better understand the problem from the patient perspective by asking the patient what she can do to help. This is the time to offer the patient a safer, quieter place on the unit, to provide support by listening, to offer reassurance about safety, and to offer any preidentified de-escalation preferences. The nurse must remain empathetic and calm, allowing the patient space and time to express her distress. This is also the time to communicate clear behavioral expectations and enlist the patient in problem solving. The nurse should not do this by telling the patient "You must ..." or "You should ...." Rather, the nurse may say: "I'd really like to help you to find a way to feel better," "You cannot leave right now," "Banging on the doors will not get you discharged," or "What else can we do that would be most helpful to you right now?" During this attempt to communicate and calm the patient, the nurse must be aware of her own nonverbal behavior and that of the patients. The nurse should be standing with a relaxed posture, watching the patient for signs of calming or escalation (Johnson & Hauser, 2001; Stokowski, 2007).

Address imminent violence. If the situation continues to escalate, and violence seems imminent, more directive action might be needed. The staff should take a team approach, with one leader assigning roles to other staff and speaking to the patient, another staff member monitoring the upset patient, and other staff securing the environment. The lead staff person should be the only person speaking to the patient at any one time. If more than one person addresses the patient, it is possible to give confusing directions, increase the stimulation, and otherwise escalate the situation further.

As staff members carry out their roles, they should keep their personal safety in mind and maintain a safe distance from the patient as much as possible. They should also make every effort to remain calm and controlled in their manner of speaking and moving around the unit. It is essential to keep the atmosphere as nonstimulating as possible in order to help everyone (staff and patients alike) stay calm.

In order to secure the environment, the first task is to segregate the target patient from other people. This can be accomplished by directing other people (including patients and visitors) to another area of the unit and engaging them in activities elsewhere. In addition to removing the "audience," the environment should be cleared of potentially harmful items. For example, chairs can be moved or sharp instruments can be put away.

When the identified staff member talks to the target patient, she should deliver comments in a calm and confident voice. Simple directions are most effective, such as "Please sit down" or "Please come with me." It may be useful to point out to the patient that he can be in control and that the staff is there to help. She can tell the patient that the staff wants to help him be in control. If medication is available by physician order, the nurse can offer the medication to him by saying, "I can give you some medication that should help you to feel calmer and in more control. Would you like me to do that?"

If it becomes evident that the patient is not responding to verbal cues and is escalating, the lead staff person may want to have a number of staff positioned to her sides. This is sometimes called "a show of strength." This gives the message that the staff will not allow violence and that the staff is ready to respond and physically stop the violence if necessary.

MIDDLE: WHEN VIOLENCE IS OCCURRING

Use Self-Defense if Necessary

If staff are unable to de-escalate the patient, he or she may behave in an aggressive way and may try to strike out at staff or other patients or destroy property. In this case, staff may need to defend themselves or physically hold the patient back from attacking another person. Staff should be trained in using techniques that will not harm a patient. For example, self-defensive techniques may include protecting one's head and midsections from a patient assault, ducking away, moving out of reach, moving the target of an anticipated strike, or blocking a blow.

Use Restraint or Seclusion as a Last Resort

Definitions. Center for Medicare & Medicaid Services (2006) provide the following definitions of seclusion and restraint. "Seclusion is the involuntary confinement of a person alone in a room or an area where the person is physically prevented from leaving. Seclusion may only be used for the management of violent or self-destructive behavior." "A physical restraint is (A) any manual method or physical or mechanical device, material or equipment that immobilizes or reduces the ability of a person to move his or her arms, legs, body or head freely; or (B) a drug or medication when it is used as a restriction to manage the person's behavior or restrict the person's freedom of movement and is not a standard treatment or dosage for the person's condition; (C) a restraint does NOT include devices, such as orthopedically prescribed devices, surgical dressings or bandages, protective helmets, or other methods that involve the physical holding of a patient for the purpose of conducting routine physical examinations or tests, or to protect the patient from falling out of bed, or to permit the patient to participate in activities without the risk of physical harm (this does not include a physical escort)" (Center for Medicare & Medicaid Services, 2006). In this chapter, we refer to a drug or medication used for restraint purposes as "chemical restraint."

Ethical and regulatory issues. Restraint and seclusion require a physician order and are regulated heavily by law and multiple regulatory bodies. Agencies will have policies and procedures in place for the use of restraint and seclusion, and these interventions are usually only acceptable when there is imminent risk of harm to self or others. Since these interventions may infringe on a patient's right to autonomy, they are never appropriate as a staff convenience or a punishment for unacceptable behavior, and a patient must be released from any restraint or seclusion when the risk of imminent harm has diminished.

Staff training. Any staff involved in restraint and/or seclusion must undergo specific training on a regular basis. The type and breadth of the training is defined by regulation (American Psychiatric Nurses Association [APNA], 2007). The Centers for Medicare and Medicaid Services, the National Association of State Mental Health Program Directors, the APNA, and the Substance Abuse and Mental Health Services Administration have all come forward with statements, white papers, and recommendations for hospitals and other organizations that care for the mentally ill to eliminate the use of restraint and seclusion through early intervention. Consequently, many health care organizations have developed a training process for all employees, which is intensive and ongoing. There are several established companies that offer training to groups or individuals. These training programs usually involve heavy emphasis on prevention or de-escalation and on learning safer techniques for restraint. There is no evidence in the literature that identifies one training program to be more effective than another. However, the literature does indicate that some kind of de-escalation training, along with staff attitudes, skill mix and workload, and various environmental factors, plays a significant role in the frequency of physical violence on an inpatient unit (Gates, Fitzwater, & Succop, 2005; McGill 2006; McPhaul & Lipscomb, 2004; National Institute for Occupational Safety and Health, 2002; Peek-Asa et al., 2009).

Risks of restraining a patient. Restraint is discouraged and heavily regulated because anytime a staff puts a hand on an agitated patient, there is potential for injury. If a patient must be immobilized by staff, a number of techniques may be employed; a common procedure is to have five staff members lower the patient to the floor, and to assign each staff member to immobilize one leg, one arm, or the head. During such a hold, the patient is at risk for positional asphyxia, especially when positioned face down on the floor (Moylan, 2009). This situation is made more dangerous when staff hold the person to the floor by kneeling or leaning on the patient's back or holding the ankles and the wrists together in a "hog-tied" position. Patients run the highest risk of asphyxia within the first 5 minutes.

Supine holds present the risk of aspiration for the patient and an increased risk of being bitten, spat upon, or kicked for staff. This hold requires the staff to monitor the patient for choking or suffocation, particularly if the patient has a decreased level of consciousness due to illness or medications. It is never acceptable for the staff to cover the patient's mouth or nose with towels or other items. The head should be held from the top or the sides, and the esophagus must be protected from pressure at all times.

Finally, during restraint, patients can also die from "excited delirium." This results from the combined effects of reduced thoracic movement, drug intoxication, and catecholamine release from exertion (Mohr & Mohr, 2000; Otahbachi, Cevik, Bagdure, & Nugent, 2010).

Risks for patients undergoing chemical restraint or patients in seclusion. None of the techniques for managing a violent patient is without risk. A person who has received medication in order to manage behavior may be at risk for orthostatic hypotension, falls, delirium, increased confusion, or overdose. A violent person in seclusion might do harm to himself while in the seclusion room.

Monitoring a patient undergoing restraint or seclusion. Monitoring a person's safety is critical at this time. Continual observation by a qualified staff member is necessary to ensure patient safety. Nurses should assess the person's level of hydration, circulation, respiratory status, skin integrity, and elimination needs at the start of the process and at minimum once every hour thereafter (APNA, 2007).

END: WHAT TO DO AFTER VIOLENCE HAS OCCURRED

A violent episode on an inpatient psychiatric unit will have an impact on the patients and the staff. The patients may feel more anxious, unsafe, or otherwise disturbed by the event. They may want to know what happened and whether it can or will happen again. They may be concerned about the staff's well-being in addition to questioning the staff's ability to keep them safe in an ongoing manner. Therefore, after establishing calm and checking for injury, the episode concludes with debriefing of the aggressive patient, followed by the other patients who witnessed the event, and debriefing for the staff. Debriefing is essential to reestablishing a therapeutic environment and maintaining positive interpersonal alliances.

Check for injury. Obviously, the first step is to make sure that the target patient, other patients, and staff were not injured. If so, medical attention should be sought immediately.

Focus on calming oneself down. The nurse should recognize that many staff members may feel agitated, anxious, angry, or otherwise upset despite an outward appearance of calm. Therefore, all staff must focus on becoming calm in order to function effectively on the unit going forward. Taking a few deep breaths, getting a glass of water, washing one's face in cold water, or if possible, taking a brief walk may prove helpful in reestablishing a sense of equilibrium.

Talk with the aggressive patient. Once the patient has become calm or in control, it is important to attempt to debrief the patient. The nurse will seek to understand: Does he know what happened? How is he feeling now? Is he okay? Is there anything that can be done to prevent this in the future? Here, it is important to discover what the patient thinks he can do and also what the staff might do. What was learned from this crisis? Are there things the staff can do to help the patient remain calm in the future?

Talk with the other patients. It is often a good idea to have a community meeting to discuss the situation. A community meeting is a gathering of patients to discuss issues of concern to the entire community (Lanza et al., 2009). A staff member can facilitate a discussion in which he gently explores how "everyone" is doing. The facilitator may ask if anyone has any concerns or feelings about the day or the event and reassure the patient population that things are in control and that treatment will continue. If there are any environmental issues (e.g., damage to the furniture or to the fire extinguisher), the facilitator may share concrete information about how this will be handled.

It is important that the other patients do not "demonize" the aggressive patient. The staff can help with this by offering statements such as, "Everyone has their own issues. Although it may be difficult to let it go, it is important that each patient concentrate on the treatment she or he is here to get, and not let outside events interfere with that goal."

Some patients may ruminate about the violent incident or become exceptionally anxious and worry that additional violence will occur. The staff should spend time with these patients, acknowledging how difficult it is to be exposed to violence, and potentially how unfair it is. The nurse can reassure the patients and acknowledge it is the responsibility of the staff to keep the patients safe. Some patients, especially those who have been victims of violence, may have a particularly difficult time when other patients are violent. If an individual patient seems to have greater difficulty getting past the event, she may need additional time to discuss the event with staff. It may be helpful to discuss it with her individually and potentially frame it as an opportunity to practice new coping skills.

Allow staff to express reactions to the event to each other and supervisors. Staff should be given time to discuss the event and their feelings about the event as soon as possible after it occurs and then again a day or two later. Staff may feel angry at the patient and wish to punish the patient for the behavior. These feelings, while expected, should be discussed because punishment has no place in a psychiatric inpatient unit.

In addition to the immediate emotional reaction the staff may have, some may experience an extended stress experience. This is especially true if there is a history of trauma. Seeking outside counsel is a good idea for a staff member who continues to be distressed, to fear returning to work, or to experience ongoing feelings of incompetence or powerlessness for a period of time after the event (Hartley, 2011). It is important to realize that violence is not the norm for most work environments and should not be considered just "part of the job" in health care settings. It is true, however, that psychiatric units and emergency rooms are considered to be the most volatile of all health care settings (Leckey, 2011).

Reporting. Every organization will have specific requirements for reporting episodes of violence. Not only will it be necessary to report the violent episode to the treatment team but there may be implications for the risk management, quality improvement, and staffing depart-ments. It is important that staff be familiar with the require-ments of the organization or agency they work for and follow all appropriate reporting procedures.

REFERENCES

American Psychiatric Nurses Association (APNA). (2007). Position statement on the use of seclusion and restraint (Original, 2000; Revised, 2007). Retrieved November 29, 2011, from http:// www.apna.org/i4a/pages/index.cfm?pageid=3728

Center for Medicare & Medicaid Services. (2006). Hospital con-ditions of participation: Patients Rights—42 CFR 482.13 (December 8, 2006). *Federal Register, 71*(236), 71427.

Clarke, D. A. B., & Griffith, P. (2010). The Broset violence check-list: Clinical utility in a secure psychiatric intensive care set-ting. *Journal of Psychiatric and Mental Health Nursing, 17*(7), 614–620.

Fluttert, F., Van Meijel, B., Van Leeuwen, M., Bjorkly, S., & Nijman, H. (2011). The development of the forensic early warning signs of aggression inventory: Preliminary findings: Toward a bet-ter managment of inpatient aggression. *Archives of Psychiatric Nursing, 25*(2), 129–137.

Gates, D., Fitzwater, E., & Succop, P. (2005). Reducing assaults against nursing home caregivers. *Nursing Research, 54*(2), 119–127.

Hartley, D. R. (2011). *Workplace violence in the healthcare setting.* Georgia: National Institute for Occupational Safety and Health. OSHA 3148–01R 2004.

Hillard, J. R. (2002). Choosing antipsychotics for rapid tranquiliza-tion in the ER. *Journal of Family Practice, 1*(4), 486–491.

Johnson, M. E., & Hauser, P. M. (2001). The practice of expert psy-chiatric nurses: Accompanying the patient to a calmer space. *Issues in Mental Health Nursing, 22*, 651–668.

Lanza, M., Rierdan, J. Forester, L., & Zeiss R. (2009). Reducing vio-lence against nurses: The violence prevention community meeting. *Issues in Mental Health Nursing, 30*(12), 745–750.

Leckey, D. (2011). Ten strategies to extinguish potentially explosive behavior. *Nursing 2011, 41*(8), 55–59.

McDermott, B. D. (2011). The predictive ability of the classifica-tion of violence risk (covr) in a forensic psychiatric hospital. *Psychiatric Services, 62*(4), 430–433.

McGill, A. (2006). Evidence-based strategies to decrease psychiatric patient assaults. *Nursing Management, 37*(11), 41–44.

McPhaul, K. M., & Lipscomb, J. A. (2004). Workplace violence in healthcare: Recognized but not regulated. *The Online Journal of Issues in Nursing, 9*(3). Retrieved May 17, 2011, from http://cms. nursingworld.org/MainMenuCategories/ANAMarketplace/ ANAPeriodicals/OLIN/TableofContents

Mohr, W. K., & Mohr, B. D. (2000). Mechanisms of injury and death proximal to restraint use. *Archives of Psychiatric Nursing, 14*(6), 285–295.

Moylan, L. B. (2009). Physical restraint in acute care psychiatry. *Journal of Psychosocial Nursing, 47*(3), 41–47.

National Institute for Occupational Safety and Health. (2002). *Violence: Occupational hazards in hospitals.* Department of Health & Human Services, Centers for Disease Control, National Institute for Occupational Safety and Health. Pub No. 2001–101.

Otahbachi, M., Cevik, C., Bagdure, S., & Nugent, K. (2010). Excited delirium, restraints and unexpected death: A review of pathogenesis. *The American Journal of Forensic Medicine and Pathology, 31*(2), 107–112.

Peek-Asa, L., Casteel, C., Veerasthpurush, A., Nocera, M., Goldmacher, S., O'Hagan, E., . . . Harrison, R. (2009). Workplace violence prevention programs in psychiatric units and facilities. *Archives of Psychiatric Nursing, 23*(2), 166–176.

Stokowski, L., (2007). Alternatives to restraint and seclusion in mental health settings: Questions and answers from psychiatric nurse experts., *Medscape Nurses: Nursing Perspectives, Retrieved May 20, 2011, from http://www.medscape.com/view article/555686*

Vaaler, A. I., Iversen, V. C., Morken, G., Flavig, J. C., Pamstierna, T., & Linaker, O. M. (2011). Short-term prediction of threatening and violent behaviour in an acute psychiatric intensive care unit based on patient and environment characteristics. *BMC Psychiatry 11*:44. Retrieved September 21, 2011, from http:// www.biomedcentral.com/1471–244X/11/44

Management of Barriers to Being Therapeutic

17

Lisa A. Uebelacker, Ellen Blair,
Cynthia Belonick, Karen Larsen, and
Mary E. Dubreuil

CHALLENGING EXPERIENCES

Like their patients, nurses suffer from frailties associated with being human. Every nurse will have unique strengths and weaknesses. Every nurse will feel more self-assured when working with certain types of patients, and less self-assured when working with others. Every nurse will have strong emotional reactions to some of her patients. In this chapter, we address some of the experiences that nurses have with patients that could make it hard for the nurse to behave in a therapeutic way, and provide some suggestions for how to cope with these experiences in a way that is clinically useful for the patient and healthy for the nurse. We address both internal experiences (thoughts and feelings occurring in relation to patients) and external experiences (patient behaviors that pose various levels of threat to the nurse's psychological or physical safety).

Challenging internal experiences. There are many beliefs about patients that the nurse may have that she will need to acknowledge and cope with in order to work effectively with a given patient. These include:

- The nurse believes that a patient is exaggerating the severity of symptoms. This is particularly relevant for the patients who are experiencing pain, or for the patients whom the nurse believes are "drug seeking," that is, seeking increasing dosages of medications such as opioids or benzodiazepines. This may have an impact on whether and how the nurse provides prn medications. Similarly, the nurse may believe that a psychotic patient is behaving bizarrely "on purpose," and the patient could (and of course should) make a choice to behave in a different way.

- The nurse does not want to care for a patient and/or does not like a patient. The patient may have been accused of or have admitted to a serious crime, such as spousal abuse, sexual abuse of a child, or murder. Other patients may behave in ways that continually violate the rights of others or appear to be taking advantage of the system. Still other patients may have some sort of other belief system that conflicts very strongly with the nurse's own beliefs or values. This could make it difficult to be professionally courteous to the patient, to be empathic with the patient, and to attend to the patient's needs.

- The nurse believes that a patient should be able to control his behavior, and is choosing not to. It may also be challenging or a problem when the nurse believes the opposite, that is, that a patient has no control over his own behavior. Both beliefs can lead to expectations about how a patient should or should not behave; these expectations may not necessarily be accurate or useful.

- The nurse believes that a patient is completely unable to make decisions for himself. This may lead to overcaring for the patients, not including patients in important conversations about their care, and not allowing the patients the maximum degree of autonomy that they are capable of having.

- The nurse believes that she is the only one who can take care of a patient. This could lead to the nurse not sharing necessary information with other team members, and feeling burdened. Further, the nurse may then not have the necessary distance to see changes in behavior that could lead to aggression or suicide. If the patient also comes to believe that only one staff member can care for her, the patient is then at risk because her preferred caregiver is not on the unit all the time.

- The nurse believes that nothing can help a given patient and that the patient's situation is hopeless. This may interfere with the nurse's actual helping behaviors, and the nurse may not try her hardest to assist this patient. If this belief is communicated to the patient in obvious or subtle ways, it could further reinforce the patient's own belief that his situation is hopeless, leading to more despair and decreased likelihood of improvement.

- The nurse notices a lot of similarities with the patient and his own life situation. This may trigger strong emotions for the nurse. For example, if the patient is similar in age and life situation (e.g., the nurse and the patient are both getting a divorce), the nurse may come to believe that "this could happen to me–I could become this debilitated." Strong similarities could also lead to the nurse spending a lot of time at work ruminating on her own problems instead of attending to patients. A strong similarity could cause the nurse to minimize the patient's problems as a way of minimizing her own problems. Finally, a strong similarity in some aspects of life could lead the nurse to assume that he knows exactly what the patient feels or needs without checking with the patient.

- The nurse really likes a patient. In some cases, the nurse could be sexually attracted to the patient. This may lead to special treatment for that particular patient. The nurse may bring in small or large gifts for the patient. The nurse could have difficulty setting appropriate boundaries or limits with the patient.

- The nurse believes that other team members are not making good choices with regard to caring for a patient. This could range from simply disagreeing with the other team member's approach to talking with the patient to other team members engaging in clear boundary violations that infringe on the patient's rights or take advantage of the patient.

These beliefs and other experiences can be associated with various intense emotional reactions for the nurse. The nurse can feel:

- angry at a particular patient for his behavior, at her colleagues for not reacting in the correct way, or at the "system" for failing a patient;
- helpless and frustrated when interventions for a particular patient do not seem to be working;
- unappreciated for his efforts;
- sad or even traumatized by the difficult life story of a given patient;
- fearful for his own safety or the safety of the patient; or
- exhausted by the intensity of the work and the associated emotions.

These emotional reactions can also lead to a nurse questioning her own decisions and global beliefs about herself. She may have thoughts such as "I am not competent," "I am not an empathic person," or even "I've gone into the wrong profession." These thoughts, in turn, can lead to a stronger emotional reaction.

Challenging external experiences. We touch on just a few here; these are experiences that range from very mild to severe crossings or violations of boundaries between nurse and patient:

- A patient asks the nurse for personal information. Common questions may include: "Are you married?" or "Where do you live?" Depending on who is asking the question and the context of the question, it may feel simply like the patient is making conversation or is experiencing normal curiosity about a person she has revealed intimate thoughts and feelings to. In other circumstances, these questions could feel threatening or invasive.

- A patient makes subtle or obvious sexual advances toward a nurse. Again, the context here will be important. A disorganized patient who is being helped with dressing and bathing may believe that, given the intimate nature of the care provided, the nurse is a significant other. Alternatively, a young patient may ask a young nurse out on a date.
- A patient is verbally abusive to a nurse—the patient yells, makes threats, swears at the nurse, or calls him names.
- A patient physically assaults a nurse.

COPING WITH CHALLENGING EXPERIENCES IN A THERAPEUTIC WAY

We offer five guiding principles for coping with these potential barriers to being therapeutic. The nurse should:

1. Acknowledge and accept her own emotions and internal reactions.
2. Acknowledge that we are all limited in our understanding of another person's (i.e., the patient's) experience.
3. Seek guidance and peer support.
4. Choose an ethical course of action.
5. Recognize the limits of his own abilities to help the patient.

Acknowledge and accept her own emotions and internal reactions. First, the nurse should examine and identify his beliefs, doubts, or concerns, as well as the associated emotions. In some cases, a negative emotion or discomfort with a patient will be the first clue that the nurse should examine her beliefs about a particular patient. It is important for the nurse to accept, without self-condemnation, that negative thoughts and emotions toward patients arise at times, and that all nurses have beliefs about patients that may turn out to be erroneous. It is also important for the nurse to accept that he may like some patients more than others. This happens with all health care professionals, from the most novice to the most experienced. Identification of a challenging situation and potential barriers to behaving therapeutically and acceptance of the nurse's internal reactions are the first steps toward actively choosing an ethical course of action with that particular patient.

Acknowledge that we are all limited in our understanding of another person's experience. In order to build his own feelings of empathy toward a patient and increase the ability to flexibly respond to the patient, the nurse will want to think about the limits of his understanding. It is hard to truly know why a patient behaves in a certain way, what type of life history brought her to the present moment, and how much "control" she has over her behavior. The issue of how much control over one's own behavior that humans have has been debated by Western philosophers for centuries.

Seek guidance and peer support. It is critical that the nurse obtain guidance from her peers and/or the physician and treatment team. Although this is particularly important when the nurse is making a decision about when or how to medicate, it is also relevant whenever a patient evokes significant negative emotions in the nurse. Guidance can range from informal discussions during the day to more structured discussion in a treatment team. "Clinical supervision" is also good context for getting feedback. "Clinical Supervision" refers to a formal, structured process of professional support. In psychiatric nursing, it is imperative to have regular supervision with an experienced nurse or other professional to discuss the feelings evoked when interacting with challenging patients. Supervision assists the nurse to understand issues associated with her practice, to gain new insights and perspectives, and to develop her knowledge and skills to improve patient and career outcomes (Hallberg, 1999). Professional nursing practice must provide the opportunity for clinical discussion that supports critical thinking and decision making. This may help the nurse to maintain a sense of identity as a caring and educated professional.

Choose an ethical course of action. Now, the nurse must choose to behave in a way that is caring and nonjudgmental and in the best interests of the patient. She will ask herself this question: "What is the best way I can help this patient move toward stabilization and decreased psychopathology?" In doing so, the nurse will keep in mind core principles of medical ethics:

- *Respect for autonomy.* This includes obtaining informed consent for treatment whenever possible, giving patients truthful information about their treatment options and other choices, supporting patient choice, and maintaining confidentiality (Butts & Rich, 2008). This can be difficult in psychiatric patients when patients' competence to make decisions is called into question and when patients' choices may differ depending on the current (and changeable) state of their disorder. However, it remains true that supporting patient autonomy to whatever extent possible is a core principle. The nurse can ask herself (and fellow team members): "What does the patient want? Do the patient and his family have the information they need to make a choice? Am I being truthful with this patient? Are there creative ways we can support patient autonomy?"
- *Nonmaleficence*, or "do no harm." This means actively avoiding negligence and any behaviors that could cause the patient harm (Butts & Rich, 2008). The nurse may ask

himself: "What can I do that will not hurt this patient? What do practice guidelines suggest? How can I make sure that my behavior is in the service of the patient rather than meeting my own or someone else's needs?"

- *Beneficence.* This refers to actively trying to work in the best interests of one's patient. The nurse will want to ask himself–and his colleagues: "How can we collaborate to do the best we can for this patient? What is the best treatment for this particular problem? How can we make sure that we are treating this patient with kindness, dignity, and respect?
- *Justice.* This is treating people fairly and without prejudice–keeping in mind that slavish adherence to rules is not the same as fair treatment, and that the "playing field" is often not level to start with. That is, different patients will need different responses because of their differing needs. However, all patients deserve and should receive the best care possible to help with the problems that brought them into the hospital.

It is crucial for the nurse to have a good understanding of ethics and be concerned with "right and wrong" as it applies to the care of each patient. The American Nurse's Association (2001) Code for Nurses states: "The nurse promotes, advocates for, and strives to protect the health, safety, and rights of the patient."

Recognize the limits of his own abilities to help the patient. Finally, the nurse should keep in mind that most of his patients have chronic problems with psychiatric illnesses and may have chronic medical problems as well. The goals of inpatient (and outpatient) treatment may be stabilization rather than a full recovery. The nurse should be aware of any needs to "cure" or "rescue" the patient and reset his goals to be more realistic and ultimately less disappointing. Although the inpatient psychiatric nurse meets his patients in the midst of a crisis, it is important to recognize that they have been using maladaptive coping mechanisms for many years. Thus, helping a patient learn new coping skills and change behavior will take time. As nurses, we will offer the best of our knowledge and our skills; however, it is truly left to the patient to accept our care, help, and concern. Even with the nurse's best efforts, the patient may choose not to accept help at this time.

REFERENCES

American Nurses Association. (2001). *Code of ethics for nurses.* Retrieved October 24, 2010, from www.nursingworld.org/codeofethics

Butts, J. B., & Rich, K. L. (2008). *Nursing ethics across the curriculum and into practice* (2nd ed.). Boston MA: Jones and Bartlett Publishers.

Hallberg, B. A. (1999). Effects of systematic clinical supervision on psychiatric nurses' sense of coherence, creativity, work-related strain, job satisfaction and view of the effects from clinical supervision: A pre-post test design. *Journal of Psychiatric Mental Health Nursing, 6*(5), 371–381.

Index

Fear
of pain, 157–158
in paranoid patients
assessment of, 192–193
interventions, 193–197
in withdrawn patients, 276
Feelings, acknowledgement
and validation of, 19, 20,
119–120
"Flight or fight" response, 27–28
Fluid intake. *See* Nutrition
Forensic Early Warning Signs of
Aggression Inventory, 364
Frustration, of patient with manic
behavior, 92–93
Functional analysis, for anger
management, 16–17
Functioning, of patient in pain
assessment of, 158–159
interventions, 159–162

Gate control theory of pain,
136–137
Gender differences, in anger
expression, 3
Generalized anxiety disorder, 30.
See also Anxiety
Goals
identification of, 354–355
setting, assistance for
patients in pain, 159–160
patients under detoxification,
229–230
Goths, 103
Groups/group therapy. *See also*
Unit-based activities
attendance, 126
for paranoid patients, 200
for patients with disorganized
behavior, 67
for substance use disorders
patients, 236
for withdrawn patients, 294
Guided imagery, 332–333

Hallucinations
in paranoid patients, 178
and suicidal risk, 244
in withdrawn patients,
275, 280, 287
Harm reduction plan, for NSSI, 126
Harm to others, risk for. *See also*
Self-harm
in patients with anger
assessment of, 6–8
interventions, 8–12
in patients with manic behavior
assessment of, 79–80
interventions, 80–82
in withdrawn patients
assessment of, 286–288
interventions, 288–290
Helplessness, 139
Home environment, for suicidal
patients, 269. *See also*
Environment; Family
interventions
Hopelessness, 377
of suicidal patients, 258–259
Hwabyung, 5
Hydromorphone, for pain
management, 151
Hygiene support
for paranoid patients, 191–192
for withdrawn patients,
283–284
Hypersexual behavior, in patients
with manic behavior
assessment of, 82–84
interventions, 84–85
Hyperventilation, 45–46
support during, 37–38

Ibuprofen (Motrin)
for pain management, 150
for patients under
detoxification, 226
and substance abuse
disorders, 209